Behavior and the Development of Representational Models of Attachment

Mary Main's groundbreaking book, unpublished until now, offers a full account of the methods she developed that revolutionized attachment research, explores her conceptual frameworks and methodologies, including the Adult Attachment Interview and coding systems, and provides essential insights into attachment theory.

The book delves into Main's innovative methods, such as the Adult Attachment Interview, the 6-year systems introducing controlling strategies, and an advanced coding system for disorganized attachment. It also includes theoretical discussions that remain highly relevant today, even as some methods are no longer in use. This work captures the depth of her contributions.

This book is indispensable for psychologists, researchers, and students of attachment theory. It is also valuable for professionals in developmental psychology, social work, and related fields seeking to understand Mary Main's revolutionary ideas and their lasting impact on attachment research.

Mary Main (deceased) was a professor of psychology emerita, University of California, Berkeley. She was the co-originator of the Adult Attachment Interview (protocol and scoring and classification system). She also collaborated in the development of many other attachment-related methods, including infant disorganized attachment and frightening/frightened behavior. Mary Main's original manuscript has been edited by Robbie Duschinsky, Erik Hesse, Kate White, and Pehr Granqvist.

Robbie Duschinsky is a professor of social science and health at the University of Cambridge and a fellow of Sidney Sussex College, Cambridge. His books include *Developments in Attachment Research* (2025) and *Cornerstones of Attachment Research* (2020).

Erik Hesse is an adjunct associate professor (retired) at the University of California, Berkeley. He collaborated in the discovery and development of methods related to "cannot classify" in the Strange Situation, and frightened/frightening parental behavior.

Kate White is a retired attachment-based psychoanalytic psychotherapist, supervisor, and member of The Bowlby Centre, London. She is the editor emerita of the journal *Attachment: New Directions in Psychotherapy and Relational Psychoanalysis*. She is currently the series editor of *The Bowlby Centre Monographs*, published by Routledge. Her publications include co-editing *Trauma and Loss: Key Texts from the John Bowlby Archive* (Routledge, 2019) with Robbie Duschinsky.

Pehr Granqvist is a professor of psychology at Stockholm University. His research spans attachment theory across the lifespan, with particular focus on attachment measurement, disorganized attachment, and applications. He has contributed widely to both empirical and theoretical advancements in the field.

Evolutions in Psychoanalysis Book Series
Series Editors
Daniel Goldin and Melvin Bronstein

Under the editorship of Melvin Bronstein and Daniel Goldin, the Evolutions in Psychoanalysis book series provides a shared space for writers who are eager to revisit formative psychoanalytical ideas in often innovative new ways. The word 'evolve' literally means 'to unroll', and the contemporary use of the latter term suggests that something new can be revealed through a process of incremental unravelling. As a definition of both the aspirations of this series and of psychoanalysis itself, this understanding exemplifies the possibility that one can take apart by creating and create by taking apart.

The volumes in this series do not represent a particular school of psychoanalytic thought, but rather comprise and encourage new voices from all schools and spaces – across time and geographical location – in the knowledge that brilliant thinkers and ideas can emerge from unforeseen places. The series does also encompass the editors' interests in how contemporary psychoanalysis intersects with society and culture at large; differing analyses of the micro-processes that take place in clinical encounters; and the influence of other disciplines – such as philosophy and infant-research – upon the field of psychoanalysis, and welcomes contributions to these and other topics.

Of critical importance to the formation of this series is its aspiration to foreground voices from marginalized ethnic groups, for the vitality and creativity they offer, which is so necessary to the field, and to continue in the direction of redress and repair for the omissions and exclusions of the past.

Practicing Psychoanalysis in Israel
Seeing Through Blindness
Gabriela Mann

Behavior and the Development of Representational Models of Attachment
Five Methods of Assessment
Mary Main
Edited by Robbie Duschinsky, Erik Hesse, Kate White, and Pehr Granqvist

For more information about this series, please visit: https://www.routledge.com/Evolutions-in-Psychoanalysis-Book-Series/book-series/EVIPS

Behavior and the Development of Representational Models of Attachment

Five Methods of Assessment

Mary Main

Edited by Robbie Duschinsky, Erik Hesse, Kate White, and Pehr Granqvist

Routledge
Taylor & Francis Group
LONDON AND NEW YORK

Designed cover image: Getty Images

First published 2027
by Routledge
4 Park Square, Milton Park, Abingdon, Oxon OX14 4RN

and by Routledge
605 Third Avenue, New York, NY 10158

Routledge is an imprint of the Taylor & Francis Group, an informa business

British Library Cataloguing-in-Publication Data
A catalogue record for this book is available from the British Library

ISBN: 978-1-032-94292-6 (hbk)
ISBN: 978-1-032-93724-3 (pbk)
ISBN: 978-1-003-56997-8 (ebk)

DOI: 10.4324/9781003569978

Typeset in Optima
by Apex CoVantage, LLC

Contents

Preface

Kate White, Pehr Granqvist, Erik Hesse, and Robbie Duschinsky

Main's contributions to attachment theory and research have been described by Van IJzendoorn and Bakermans-Kranenburg (1997, p. 138) as a "revolutionary shift." Jeremy Holmes (2009, p. 4) characterized her work as the start of attachment research "Phase 2" and Cowan et al. (2023) described Mary as a "towering and path-breaking figure." Central elements of this revolution were the conceptual and methodological innovations Main developed in the late 1980s, and wrote up as the present book in 1986. John Bowlby (1990) wrote to Sonia Monteiro de Barros: "I wonder if you are following Mary Main's recent work? . . . She has a book in press with Cambridge University Press which will be very remarkable."

Yet sadly, this book remained unpublished until now. Those who have wanted to understand Main's work have been reliant on her published articles and chapters. The consequence of this has been that the details of her most important research methods have remained inaccessible to all but a few who received personal manuscripts from Main in her lifetime. This has contributed to misapprehensions of the nature of Main's contributions to attachment theory and research, and the location and extent of their value (see Hesse, 2016; Duschinsky, 2025).

Each chapter in this remarkable book is devoted to a different research method developed by Mary and her colleagues and designed to assess attachment organization in toddlers, young children, and adults.

The breadth and depth of this book are startling.

This is a book of methods for the identification and classification of human attachment organization as it is encountered in infant behavior; in adult autobiographical memory; in children's family drawings; in child–parent discourse; and in the behavioral response of 6-year-olds to reunion with the parent following an hour's separation in the laboratory.

The volume begins with Main's own foundational essay, "Behavior and the Development of Representational Models of Attachment," which articulates the core theoretical integration that would shape much of her later work.

In "Procedures for Identifying Infants as Disorganized/Disoriented During the Ainsworth Strange Situation," co-authored with Judith Solomon, we see the introduction of the now widely adopted Disorganized classification – a concept that has expanded and enriched our understanding of attentional strategies as they emerge in childhood.

"The Adult Attachment Interview," co-authored with Carol George and Nancy Kaplan, marks a turning point in attachment research, extending the focus beyond infancy and offering a method to explore adults' states of mind with respect to attachment.

This is further developed in "An Adult Attachment Classification System," co-authored with Ruth Goldwyn (in 1986) and subsequently with Erik Hesse (in 2003), which outlines the methodology for evaluating adult discourse, particularly the construct of "coherence of mind" – a term now central in both research and clinical contexts.

In "Relationship Representation in Child–Parent Discourse: Instructions for Classifying Seven Central Patterns," written with Amy Strage, we see an innovative application of discourse analysis to the developing child, foreshadowing much later work on narrative and representation in child psychology.

The theme of representation continues in "Instructions for the Classification of Children's Family Drawings in Terms of Representation of Attachment," with Nancy Kaplan, where visual narrative becomes a window into the internal working models of children.

Finally, "Assessments of Child–Parent Attachment at Six Years of Age," co-authored with Jude Cassidy, reflects a developmental extension of the Strange Situation methodology, providing tools for assessing attachment beyond the toddler years.

Together, these chapters reveal the breadth and depth of Mary Main's intellectual legacy. They show us a researcher deeply committed to empirical precision, theoretical clarity, and the ethical imperative of understanding the child's and the adult's inner worlds. Through rigorous observation and careful analysis, Main has given us language and structure for phenomena that were once only intuited.

It should be noted by readers that this is a historical document, now essentially of theoretical and historical relevance rather than a how-to guide for conducting assessments of attachment. At the time of writing, these coding systems were still being developed. Indeed, the final Adult Attachment Interview and Six-Year Assessment have evolved considerably and look quite different from the early versions from 1986. For those interested in training on these coding systems, see https://mainattachment.org

Nonetheless, we hope the reader, like us, sees value in having access to the 1986 manuals all together: as an insight into Main's methodological and theoretical innovations, and as a provocation to consider and reflect on her legacy of transformation in attachment theory and research. We hope this collection not only honors Mary Main's extraordinary contributions but also invites continued dialogue and innovation. Her work challenges us to look beyond the observable, to attend to meaning beneath behavior, and to remain open to the complexity of human attachment across the lifespan.

Introduction

Each of the methods presented in this volume has been developed over a period of several years, utilizing a sample of white, middle-class families residing in the Bay Area of California (described in Chapter 1). With the single exception of the deliberate, gradual development and refinement of a method for distinguishing infants who do not fit into the A, B, C attachment classification system developed by Mary Ainsworth ("D" infants, see Main & Weston, 1981; Main & Solomon, 1986; this volume), not one of the methods presented in this volume was developed deliberately as a method. Each instead is the consequence of our attempt to address an issue involving either (1) the coherence of behavior across time, for example, the predictability of sixth-year from first-year reunion behavior; (2) the way in which the adult's internal working model of her own attachment relationships is related to the infant's attachment organization as classified in the Ainsworth Strange Situation (Ainsworth et al., 1978); or (3) the way that cognitive and language mechanisms come to participate in the preservation of relationships and their internal representations.

Presenting our methods as discoveries, then, the simplest is certainly that, in a white middle-class sample of intact families such as ours, sixth-year reunion behavior can be predicted from first-year reunion behavior. Indeed, our hit-rate for prediction of attachment categories across the five-year period (84%) is almost identical to the hit-rate found in previous studies that have simply conducted the Ainsworth Strange Situation twice over a six-month or eight-month period in infancy (Main & Cassidy, this volume). We have also discovered that the composition of children's drawings can be predicted from their early attachment classifications (Kaplan & Main, 1986; this volume), as can their discourse with the parent (Strage & Main, 1985; this volume). Predictions of discourse patterns are particularly striking. In a group of 66 transcripts, we achieved 67% accuracy in predicting seven attachment sub-groups (see the following section for a description of the attachment sub-classifications).

Finally, we have found that an infant's attachment classification to a particular parent corresponds to the parent's adult attachment classification, as determined from a study of transcripts of an Adult Attachment Interview devised by George, Kaplan, and Main (1985 and this volume). Verbatim transcriptions of this interview permit a judge to assess the adult's overall "internal working model" of attachment, that is, the way in which the individual is currently organizing her thoughts and feelings with respect to her own attachment history. It is this internal adult organization which is reflected directly in the organization of the infant's response to separation and to leave-taking. Specifically, a child who is judged, for example, *secure* with mother in infancy is most likely to have a mother judged *secure/autonomous* in terms of her own internal representations.

The presentation of these discoveries was withheld until each had been replicated in at least one independent laboratory. Each replication study has involved the use of the methods presented here and comparisons of outcomes to infant Strange Situation behaviors as classified in the second laboratory. It is the work undertaken in these laboratories which has given me confidence that these methods do actually represent attachment-related aspects of human mental organization, and will therefore be useful to others.

The immediate audience for this volume will be, of course, the growing body of individuals interested in the study of attachment. Some workers will simply be glad to have available for the first time methods of assessing individual differences in attachment organization in childhood and in adulthood. Others will welcome a revision of their present Strange Situation codings in which, no doubt, some infants presently coded as B (secure) but who are in fact "D" infants (disorganized) are behaving like insecure infants in other settings. As of the time of this writing, many laboratories have in fact already re-coded their Strange Situation tapes using the new "disorganized/disoriented" (D) classification presented here and elsewhere (Main & Solomon, 1986). It is clear that both the Adult Attachment Classification System and the technique for analysis of children's drawings can be used in the clinical setting, not only in making initial assessments of one's patients or prospective patients but also in ongoing and follow-up assessments throughout the course of therapy. Several projects of this type are underway, in psychiatry and clinical psychology, as well as in developmental psychology, involving the Adult Attachment Interview and the new method of assessment of children's family drawings.

In my view, however, the audience for which these methods will be useful is much wider. Consideration of the ways in which dyads and individuals seek actively to preserve their mental or dyadic attachment organization suggests at once a multitude of new experiments involving discourse, pragmatics, perception, and memory. (See Main et al. (1985) for suggestions for some specific future experiments.)

The remainder of this section is devoted to a brief historical overview of the field of attachment. This discussion is provided to give readers outside the field of developmental psychology some sense of orientation as they approach the methods presented in this volume.

In a series of volumes published between 1969 and 1980, the London family psychiatrist John Bowlby founded a new field of scientific and psychiatric inquiry, which he termed *attachment* (Bowlby, 1969, 1973, 1980). Attachment theory took as its roots both naturalistic and laboratory observations of non-human animals (especially, primates) and a new understanding of environmentally stable behavior patterns (formerly, "instinctive" behavior patterns) as being organized in terms of "control systems."

Bowlby's essential hypothesis was that, over the course of the first years of life, human beings, like other ground-living primates, develop an "attachment behavioral system." This is a system of instinctively guided behavior patterns, which become focused upon one or a few central, parental figures (attachment figures). The "attachment behavioral system" is presumed to have evolved through natural selection. It has the biological function of ensuring that the infant, through its active proximity-seeking or through signaling behavior (e.g., crying), maintains itself in a position where an attachment figure is accessible. This propensity towards active proximity-keeping is expected because, in the environment of evolutionary adaptedness, the young ground-living primate does not survive unless kept in the company of others – and specifically, in most species, in the company of the mother. Thus, proximity to the attachment figure is the *sine qua non* for the young primate's survival.

Although the attachment behavioral system is presumed to be continually active (alert to the present and likely state of accessibility and/or proximity of one or a few attachment figures), attachment behavior is not expected to be activated when the infant is held by the mother, or when mother is calm, nearby, and obviously ready to attend to her infant if needed. The infant of over 8 months is then expected to be occupied with exploration and play, its other major concerns. When, however, the infant is alarmed or stressed in any way, whether stemming from sudden threatening changes in the environment, illness, or the possibility or reality of mother's sudden leave-taking, the attachment behavioral system is expected to be activated at higher levels. The infant is then expected to seek the mother through attempts to pursue her, or else by signaling for her (crying).

Bowlby proposed this behavioral system to be of equal import to the sexual behavioral system in explaining major aspects of both normal and anomalous forms of human behavior. In particular, Bowlby used the new theory to explain the effects of long, stressful separations from parents – separations such as hospitalizations in which the child was offered neither parental visiting nor substitute parental figures – upon young toddlers. While these and comparable experiences were in no sense genuinely physically harmful to young children, they were observed to cause changes in the personality. Bowlby suggested that these changes occurred because the attachment behavioral system was not designed to develop or function in circumstances which depart so widely from those which the infant would meet with in the environment of evolutionary adaptedness. The chief changes identified in toddlers who had undergone long, stressful separations from all attachment figures were two syndromes well known to clinicians working with adult patients. These were:

1. A syndrome of *detached, affectionless* behavior, in which feeling for others appeared peculiarly absent, and especially for others who had previously been or were now expected to be attachment figures. I shall call this Pattern A.
2. A syndrome of *anxious, clinging* behavior, often combined with hostility, in which the individual suffered continual distress and concern with the whereabouts or emotional accessibility of others. I shall call this Pattern C.

Bowlby's theory was introduced to the United States through the pioneering work of a developmental psychologist, Mary Ainsworth. Ainsworth had worked with Bowlby in London, and had subsequently spent a year in Uganda observing Ganda families, and specifically, the development of infant–mother attachment within those families. Once settled in Baltimore, she determined to see whether attachment behaviors developed and became organized and focused on the mother in the same way in Baltimore as previously observed in Uganda. Her observations were extensive. She and her assistants made between 16 and 21 4-hour home visits to 26 infant–mother dyads throughout the first year of the infant's life. She ended this longitudinal study with a brief observation of infant responses to mother's leave-taking and return in a strange environment, now known as the Ainsworth Strange Situation (Ainsworth & Wittig, 1969; Ainsworth et al., 1978).

In conducting separation-and-reunion observations in the laboratory setting, Ainsworth intended only to demonstrate Bowlby's general points regarding the way in which infants of this age will respond to a strange environment in the mother's presence, then to the mother's leave-takings, and then to her two returns. Since none of the sample infants had experienced major separations from their mothers, she expected all infants to behave as follows (Ainsworth, personal communication, May, 1984):

1. When mother and infant were alone in the room in the first episode of the observation, the mother's presence was expected to override any distress the infant might otherwise have experienced in response to the strange environment. The infant was expected to spend this episode exploring the toys.
2. By the mother's second leave-taking (if not the first), attachment behavior was expected to take precedence over exploratory behavior, and the infant was expected to show distress and seek the mother.
3. When the mother returned, the infant was expected to actively seek proximity to the mother, maintain contact with her for a minute or so, and then, reassured once more regarding her presence, the infant was expected to return to play.

A small majority of the infants (13/23) seen in Ainsworth's Strange Situation did in fact behave approximately as she expected. A substantial minority, however, did not. Six ignored the mother's leave-taking and actively avoided her upon reunion (these were later classified as "A" babies). Four were distressed and anxious even in the mother's presence, and could not be comforted nor led to return to play upon her return (these were later classified as "C" babies). Since Ainsworth had narrative records of a full year of infant–mother interaction available, she determined to return to a study of these records to see whether the peculiar patterns of detached *avoidance* (A) and anxious *resistance* (C) could be explained.

Ainsworth's analysis of her home narrative records revealed that each of the three patterns of infant reaction to the Strange Situation procedure was associated with different kinds of experiences with mother throughout the first year of life. Specifically:

Group B. The infants who had shown distress at leave-taking, proximity-seeking upon reunion, and then, comforted, returned to play had mothers who were sensitive to their signals and accepting of their attachment behavior throughout the first year of life.

Group A. The infants who showed no distress at mother's leave-taking, then actively avoided the mother on reunion, had mothers who actively rejected the infant's attachment behavior (and particularly, physical contact with the infant) throughout the first year of life. Some of the mothers of "A" infants stated directly that they disliked them or wished that they had never had them.

Group C. The infants who showed fear and distress even when mother was present, extreme distress at her absence, anger at her reunion, and an inability thereafter to be settled or returned to play had mothers who were insensitive to their signals throughout the first year of life. These mothers were likely to be extremely inaccessible at times (one mother left her infant alone in its room for two weeks, going in only briefly to feed it), or else were extremely interfering (one mother attempted to teach her infant to walk at six months). At times, the mothers of the "C" infants could be warm, but they were inconsistent.

In a later article, Ainsworth further described the patterning of infant Strange Situation behavior not only in terms of the A, B, and C groups described earlier but also in terms of sub-group patterns. Thus, for example, she described two kinds of "insecure-avoidant" (Group A) infant responses to the Strange Situation, A1 (extremely avoidant) and A2 (moderately avoidant), and she described three sub-patterns of "secure" response: B1, B2, and B3. Pattern B3 was the prototypically secure pattern described earlier. The B3 infant showed neither avoidance nor resistance to the mother upon reunion and, once having established contact on his own initiative, returned to play. Both B1 and B2 infants showed some resemblance to A infants in showing some avoidance, but the overall patterning was substantially different.

Studies of interaction in the home situation showed further that *particular patternings of infant–mother interaction lay behind the sub-groups as well as the major groups* identified within the Strange Situation. Thus, for example, mothers of the A1 infants had been rejecting of infant attachment behavior as well as extremely interfering in the home situation, while mothers of A2 infants had been rejecting and ignoring rather than interfering. The Strange Situation sub-groups were also represented in the infant's use of the mother as a "secure base" for exploration and play in the home environment. The B3 sub-group infants – judged most secure with mother in terms of the Strange Situation – showed a particularly easy, integrated balance between exploration of the home environment and returns to mother.

Ainsworth's work concerning individual differences in infant attachment organization gained especially wide acceptance following papers published by Waters (1978) and by Sroufe and Waters (1977). Waters studied a sample of 50 Minnesota infants and their mothers in the Strange Situation at 12 months and again at 18 months of age. Infants were assigned at both ages to Ainsworth's major (A, B, C) classifications and sub-classifications (which now included a fourth group B sub-category, B4). Judges at each age period were, of course, blind to the infant's behavior at the other age period.

Waters found the overall patterning of the infant's response to the mother in the Strange Situation was virtually identical at 12 and at 18 months in terms of A, B, C classifications. Moreover, 30 out of the 50 infants fell in the same one of the eight attachment *sub-groups* at the two time periods (for example, the two infants sub-classified as B1 at 12 months were classified as B1 again at 18 months of age). With these findings as well as the basic foundations of Ainsworth's position in mind, Sroufe and Waters (1977) together wrote a paper on "attachment as an organizational construct." Variables such as "minutes spent in crying," or "minutes spent touching mother" had not been found stable in Water's study, whereas the overall patterning of behavior as discovered by Ainsworth and backed by her home observations had. Sroufe and Waters stressed a point which had also been emphasized previously by Ainsworth: Behaviors of many types can serve a similar function (for example, both freezing and fleeing can be responses to fright). This interchangeability of actual behaviors shown in the service of a particular function can be missed when the researcher simply counts up the occurrence of phenotypically similar behavior patterns but can be readily recognized by the worker who, searching for overall patterning, utilizes classification. Following Sroufe and Waters' papers, the Ainsworth classification system became recognized as a major research tool. While relatively little further attention was paid to sub-groups, research involving the A, B, C's of attachment began to flourish.

It is obvious that, given the extraordinary stability of attachment organization found in Waters' study, a first issue to be settled was whether such stability was not due to constitutionally determined differences, which had nothing to do with the infant's experience with its attachment figure. If this was the case, however, then a given infant should have the same classification with mother as with father, when seen in the Strange Situation on two different occasions (with each parent). Studies in four independent laboratories have now shown that a given infant's "attachment classification (A, B, C)" to mother is independent of its classification with father (see Bretherton, 1985, for a review of these studies).

Over the past 8 years, the number of studies involving assessments of individual difference in attachment organization (through the Ainsworth Strange Situation) has increased almost geometrically. A number of investigators (including Klaus and Karin Grossmann of West Germany) have found it possible to replicate Ainsworth's finding of differences in the "sensitivity and responsiveness" of mothers of Group B vs. Groups A and C infants in the home situation (see Bretherton, 1985, for a review of these studies). Several follow-up studies of the nursery school and kindergarten behavior of children judged secure versus insecure with mother in infancy have been conducted, some involving a Berkeley sample (Waters et al., 1979); some involving a white, middle-class Minnesota sample (Arend et al., 1979); and some involving a Minnesota poverty sample (Sroufe, 1983). Most, but not all investigations in attachment have simply compared the follow-up behavior (or mothering experiences) of secure (B) versus insecure (A and C) babies (Sroufe, 1983, is a significant exception). In each of these studies, children judged secure with mother in infancy have been found to be functioning with greater competence and/or ego-resilience and/or to show more "positive" affect in the new peer settings.

A review of the remainder of studies involving use of the Ainsworth Strange Situation is beyond the scope of this Introduction. Almost all have been successful and, at minimum, have shown that infants judged secure in the Ainsworth Strange Situation have mothers whose behavior is judged more favorable than infants judged insecure in the Strange Situation, or that the secure infants themselves have been judged to be more sociable, happy, or competent either before or some years following the 12-month Ainsworth Strange Situation.

References

Bowlby, J. (1990). *Attachment and loss: Vol. 3. Loss: Sadness and depression*. Basic Books.

Cowan, P., Cowan, C.P., & Weinstein, R. (2023). Remembering Mary Main. https://psychology.berkeley.edu/news/remembering-mary-main

Duschinsky, R. (2025). Mary Main: Portrait and tribute. *Attachment & Human Development, 27*, 156–189.

Hesse, E. (2016). The adult attachment interview: Protocol, method of analysis, and selected empirical studies: 1985–2015. In J. Cassidy & P.R. Shaver (Eds.), *Handbook of Attachment: Theory, Research, and Clinical Applications* (pp. 553–597). Guilford.

Holmes, J. (2009). *Exploring in Security: Towards an Attachment-Informed Psychoanalytic Psychotherapy*. Routledge.

Van IJzendoorn, M.H., & Bakermans-Kranenburg, M.J. (1997). Intergenerational transmission of attachment: A move to the contextual level. In L. Atkinson & K.J. Zucker (Eds.), *Attachment and Psychopathology* (pp. 135–170). Guilford.

1 Behavior and the Development of Representational Models of Attachment

Mary Main

This is a book of methods for the identification and classification of human attachment organization as it is encountered in infant behavior; in adult autobiographical memory; in children's family drawings; in child–parent discourse; and in the behavioral response of the 6-year-old to reunion with the parent following an hour's separation in the laboratory. The aim of this introductory chapter is to assist the reader in using and interpreting these methods. It is assumed that the reader is familiar with both the theory of attachment as developed by John Bowlby (Bowlby, 1969, 1973, 1980) and the discovery of and description of individual differences in infant attachment organization made by Mary Ainsworth (Ainsworth & Wittig, 1969; Ainsworth et al., 1971; Ainsworth et al., 1978).

To this point in time, the notion of classification of individuals in terms of attachment organization has been confined to infancy, and specifically to infant responses to the Ainsworth Strange Situation, an observational procedure involving parent and infant in two brief separations and reunions within the laboratory setting. Examination of infant responses to the parent's return during this procedure permits classification of infants in one of four major "attachment categories." The classifications are based largely upon the way in which the infant responds to reunion with the parent following these brief leave-takings. These four classifications of infant reaction may be very briefly described as *insecure-avoidant* (Group A – the infant actively avoids and ignores the parent); *secure* (Group B – the infant actively seeks proximity or interaction with the parent, then returns to play); *insecure-resistant* (Group C – the infant both seeks and resists the parent, and/or refuses to be settled); and *insecure-disorganized/disoriented* (Group D – the infant exhibits a diverse array of conflict behaviors described by Main and Solomon (1986); this volume). Figures 1.1–1.4 present four slightly more extensive descriptions of these four major categories of infant reaction.

DOI: 10.4324/9781003569978-1

The Ainsworth Strange Situation: *Insecure-avoidant*. The infant actively avoids and ignores the parent on reunion, looking away, turning away, and moving away if the parent pursues. The infant shows little distress throughout the situation, simply remaining pre-occupied with toys. May be relatively friendly to stranger.

The Adult Attachment Interview: *Dismissing of attachment*. The adult dismisses the importance and influence of attachment-related feelings, experiences, and memories. Her parents are typically described as excellent parents, but supportive memories are absent, or seem instead to suggest experiences of rejection. The adult may describe herself as strong.

Child–Parent Discourse at Six: *Restricted discourse*. Discourse is minimal and impersonal. There are frequent pauses between adult and child conversational turns. Topics are limited to objects and activities, and are not carried forward. The parent is in control of the conversation, but her questions tend to be rhetorical questions, yes/no answer questions, or test questions.

Family Drawings at Six: *Cheerful invulnerability*. Typically, all figures are drawn smiling. Postures are relatively stiff, with little individuation. Arms may be missing, or are placed in positions unsuitable for embracing. The smiling figures do not seem meaningfully related to one another or affected by one another and may float above the ground.

Video-taped Parent–Child Reunions at Six: *Insecure-avoidant*. The child minimizes and restricts opportunities for interaction with parent on reunion, looking and speaking only briefly and as required. She remains occupied with toys or activities. At extremes, she will subtly increase physical distance from the parent, with a rationale such as retrieving a toy.

Figure 1.1 "Pattern A" attachment organization

The Ainsworth Strange Situation: *Secure*. The infant may or may not show distress at separation. However, she seeks interaction, proximity, and/or physical contact with the parent upon reunion. She is readily soothed by the parent after distress and returns to play. She shows definite preference for parent over stranger.

The Adult Attachment Interview: *Secure/Autonomous*. The interview is coherent, that is, analysis of the text does not lead the judge to different conclusions than those that have been presented. The adult regards attachment-related experiences as influential but seems relatively independent and objective. There appears to be little idealization of the parents. The subject seems at ease with imperfection in the self and others. Attachment-related experiences may have been favorable or harsh. If harsh, the subject is thoughtful.

Figure 1.2 "Pattern B" attachment organization

Child–Parent Discourse at Six: *Fluent discourse.* Discourse has the characteristics of fluent dialogue. Few or no ignored conversational overtures by parent or child, and no long pauses except between topics. Questions appear to be genuine. Both parties may persist in moving topics forward.

Family Drawings at Six: *Rational and Realistic.* Within the level permitted by the child's skill, the drawing is realistic. Figures are grounded, centered, individuated, and often drawn with arms extended in an embracing posture. Figures suggest movement. Real-world elements are often present.

Video-taped Parent–Child Reunions at Six: *Secure.* The child initiates conversation and pleasant interaction with the parent on reunion, or is highly responsive to parent's own initiations. The child may subtly move into proximity to the parent, usually with rationale such as seeking a toy. The child is calm.

Figure 1.2 (Continued)

The Ainsworth Strange Situation: *Insecure-resistant.* The infant may be distressed even prior to separation, perhaps at entrance of stranger. Following separation, the infant's high distress is not effectively soothed by parent. Infant may seek proximity and contact, then resist it. She shows subtle to overt anger.

The Adult Attachment Interview: *Pre-occupied with early attachment relationships.* The adult appears confused, incoherent, and unobjective, seeming unable to move beyond a sense of self as enmeshed in and influenced by early relationships. Subject either accepts this state passively, or expresses strong anger. Subject may be unconvincingly analytical in speaking of her past experiences. Parents may have demanded care, or criticized and called for attempts to please. Subject may bring up irrelevant topics during the interview.

Child–Parent Discourse at Six: (*Rules not fully developed*).

Family Drawings at Six: *Vulnerability.* The family tends to be drawn as either huge (filling the page) or extremely small (perhaps in page corner). Family members tend either to be in extreme proximity (perhaps embracing), or separated by barriers, for example, child and parents on separate sides of a house. Emphasis on soft parts (belly, belly-button), and facial features (huge eyes/nostrils).

Video-taped Parent–Child Reunion at Six: *Insecure-ambivalent.* The child appears to be pretending to have a secure relationship with the parent and/or to exaggerate dependent (baby) status. She may seek proximity or contact, but show some ambivalence, for example, lying on parent's lap while wriggling uncomfortably. She is moderately avoidant with subtle signs of hostility.

Figure 1.3 "Pattern C" attachment organization

The Ainsworth Strange Situation: *Disorganized/Disoriented.* Infant shows strong conflict behaviors indicating either disorganization (e.g., approaching parent with head averted) or disorientation (e.g., stilling or freezing movement). Infant is unclassifiable within the A, B, C system.

The Adult Attachment Interview: *Lack of resolution of mourning for attachment figures.* Speech regarding attachment figures lost through death indicates lack of resolution of mourning, often in terms of (a) irrational thought processes, or (b) entrance into a relatively disoriented state of mind. (Physical or sexual abuse by parents may also be related to the "D" pattern).

Child–Parent Discourse at Six: *Dysfluent.* Stumbling and false starts by both parent and child. Child frequently addresses parent with imperatives, while parent addresses child with questions. Parent responds passively to child's steering of the conversation, that is, does not elaborate or add to the topic.

Family Drawings at Six: *Irrational.* Usually, either (a) disorganization of elements, as scratching-out and re-starts, or (b) addition of unexpected elements to the drawing or omission of expected elements, as, standing family members on a row of hearts, or putting only one eye in a head presented full-face. The overall effect of the drawing may be ominous, or over-bright.

Video-taped Parent–Child Reunion at Six: *Controlling of parent.* Child seems to attempt to control and direct the parent's behavior, either through punitive behavior (embarrassing or humiliating the parent), or over-bright/caregiving behavior. In some (rare) cases, relationship instead seems sexualized, or simply still unclassifiable.

Figure 1.4 Disorganization of attachment (D)

Observations in the home setting have shown that infants judged A, B, or C in terms of their response to reunion with the mother during the Strange Situation have experienced differing patterns of infant–mother interaction. The most extensive observations collected to date are those of Mary Ainsworth (Ainsworth et al., 1971), who observed 23 infant–mother dyads in the home situation (approximately 80 hours per dyad) over the first year of life prior to the 12-month Strange Situation assessment. She found that, as compared to infants judged insecure-avoidant (A) or insecure-resistant (C) in the Strange Situation, infants judged secure (B) had mothers who were responsive to their signals and communications in the home setting, and who were accepting of the infant's attachment behavior. This finding has now been replicated by several investigators (see Bretherton, 1985, for summary). In addition, Ainsworth found that infants judged insecure-avoidant had mothers who, in the home, were relatively rejecting, and specifically rejecting of physical contact. Infants judged insecure-resistant had mothers who were inconsistent, and either inaccessible for long periods of time or highly interfering (Ainsworth et al., 1978).

Given the dependence of the infant's reaction to the parent's return in the laboratory upon the infant's history of interaction with that particular caregiver, it is not surprising that studies have consistently shown independence of a given infant's A, B, or C "attachment classification" to mother and to father (see Bretherton, 1985, again for summary). The "D" category has also been found to be independent across mothers and fathers (Main & Solomon, 1986).

The methods presented here rest upon a series of completed studies, some reported in a series of recent papers (Main et al., 1985; Main & Solomon, 1986; Main & Cassidy, 1988; Main & Hesse, 1990), with other reports still in progress. We have discovered:

1. that a given parent's mental organization with respect to attachment is highly correspondent (similar) to the organization of the infant's attachment to that parent as observed in the Ainsworth Strange Situation. More specifically, assessment of a discussion of the parent's autobiographical history obtained through an Adult Attachment Interview (George et al., this volume) reveals four (A, B, C, D) categories of adult mental representation with respect to attachment, categories which are analogous to the four categories of infant Strange Situation behavior. Moreover, the infant's attachment classification reflects the parent's adult attachment classification, such that adults classified A in terms of the Adult Attachment Interview have infants classified A when seen with them in the Strange Situation, parents classified B have infants classified B, etc. In addition:
2. the infant's A, B, C, or D attachment classification is highly predictive of the kind of drawings which she will make of her family at six; the kind of discourse which she and her parent will engage in upon reunion as assessed sheerly from transcripts; and the child's (largely non-verbal) expressive behavior toward the parent within the reunion situation. Drawings, discourse, and non-verbal behavior are again classified in terms of A, B, C, D equivalent systems.

These discoveries present, in my view, a new level of evidence supporting the notion of structure, coherence, and predictability in behavior. The hit-rates for parent to infant (major) classifications, and for infant to sixth-year classifications, have been surprisingly strong (from 72% to 84% for the major attachment categories), and each finding has now been replicated in other, independent laboratories (as described in the following section). What is meant specifically by hit-rate is the correspondence in classification between parent and infant, or infant and 6-year-old, such that, for example, the A adult classification is associated specifically with the A infant classification, which in turn is associated specifically with the A-equivalent classifications of children's drawings, reunion behavior, and discourse.

At the very least, what can be made of these results is that the individual differences in attachment organization, first discovered by Ainsworth in infant reactions to the parent in a stressful environment, are confined neither to infancy nor to behavioral reactions to the leave-taking and return of an attachment figure. Rather, what is classified in terms of the infant's non-verbal response to the parent within the Ainsworth Strange Situation can be classified equally well when the adult speaks of and evaluates her autobiographical memories of attachment-related events, or as the 6-year-old constructs a drawing of her family. Indeed, it seems that what is being identified through these classification systems – whether they deal with spoken autobiographies, drawings, infant behavior, or discourse – is nothing less than a set of *general, relatively stable, and coherent categories of mental organization shaped through individual experiences and representations of attachment.*

The implications of these discoveries, however, go well beyond the recognition that four or more similar attachment categories can now be identified by several means, at several ages, and in several modalities. The fact that significant aspects of adult mental process are reflected so exactingly in infant non-verbal behavior –, that an adult judged dismissing of attachment has an infant judged avoidant of her as an attachment figure – suggests an entirely new specificity of linkage between the mind of one person (the parent) and the behavior of another. The parent's conceptualization of her history as inferred through spoken memories and the evaluation of those memories becomes reflected in the behavior of her infant, and specifically in the security or any of three distinct types of insecurity of her infant's attachment to her.

In addition, the fact that attachment relationships seen in infancy predict drawing, discourse, and expressive behavior toward the parent at 6 years of age suggests at once that *the preservation of relationships of particular types involves the participation of cognitive mechanisms, which include not only language usage but also perception and, in all probably, the organization of memory.* This point has been discussed at greater length earlier (Main et al., 1985).

The remainder of this chapter is devoted to a discussion of the development of each of the five methods of assessment presented in this volume.

Five Methods of Assessment

Each method of assessment was developed initially through study of a sample of white, middle-class families residing in the Bay Area of California. In the first stage of the study, infants were observed in the Strange Situation with the mother at 12 months of age, and at 18 months with the father. Five years later, 40 families returned to the laboratory, where the Adult Attachment Interview (described in the following section) was administered to each parent while the child was engaged in a number of assessments with the examiner, including a family drawing. Following approximately an hour's separation, parents were told that the assessments were over, and the mother (father) returned to the room, followed three minutes later by the father (mother).

The Bay Area Social Development Project sample was deliberately selected to enable us to study the nature and development of attachment relationships relatively unaffected by constitutional difficulties on the part of the infant; major separations from parents; divorce; or major illness on the part of either parent or child (see Main & Weston, 1981; Main et al., 1985, for a full description of sample characteristics). All of these are factors, which can potentially affect the organization of an infant's or child's attachment from sources other than the interactions which take place between the attachment figure and the child. For example, a child who has enjoyed harmonious interactions with a parent throughout the first year of life can become temporarily insecure with respect to that parent on the basis of a stressful hospitalization, even though there has been no change in the real interactions (relationship) with the parent. Our aim was to discover the transformations which occur in relationships and in relationship representations over time, without interference from sources outside of the relationship.

The five methods of assessment presented begin with the method developed for determining that an infant is disorganized and/or disoriented ("D") during the Ainsworth Strange Situation (or during another mildly stressful situation in which the infant is seen with the parent, see Main & Weston, 1981; Wartner, 1987). This method is the logical starting point, because it is only when infants showing disorganized behavior are recognized and separated from infants in the three traditional categories – and especially, are distinguished as infants inappropriate for placement in the "secure" category – that sharp predictions and associations can be made in other settings.

The Adult Attachment Interview and the Adult Attachment Classification System are presented next, in part because this forms the most radical leap from infancy. In addition, it will give the reader familiar with the Strange Situation but unfamiliar with the adult category system an opportunity to begin to develop a more general sense of what representations and experiences lie behind the categories. This should be helpful in moving next to the analysis of child–parent discourse, which, like the adult attachment classification, is based entirely upon speech transcripts. A radical change in the material examined is made when the analysis of children's family drawings is presented.

The assessment of reunion between the 6-year-old and her parent as based largely on her expressive, video-taped, non-verbal behavior is presented in conclusion. The other methods we have utilized to assess the organization of attachment may lack immediacy for observers trained to date exclusively in the analysis of video-taped infant Strange Situation behavior. This final method may seem both more immediately accessible and more familiar.

Inter-judge reliability for the five methods described in the following section ranges from 76% to 85%.

Identifying Infants as Disorganized/Disoriented

Five years ago, we reported that a substantial proportion of seemingly insecure, middle-class infants seen in the Ainsworth Strange Situation could not be satisfactorily classified using the traditional, "A, B, C" classification system. Seen in a separate setting, these infants showed more conflict behaviors than other infants. These infants were therefore set apart, and temporarily identified simply as insecure-unclassifiable (Main & Weston, 1981).

At the same time, investigators working with several maltreatment samples were also setting aside infants whom they considered unclassifiable (e.g., Egeland & Sroufe, 1981a, 1981b; Gaensbauer & Harmon, 1982). In many cases, the only alternative (or forced) classification for these infants would have been "secure." Given that the "secure" infant had been maltreated, this classification did not fit well with the investigator's knowledge of its history (see Main & Solomon, 1986, for a review of these studies).

Over the past 3 years, a close study of the particulars of the Strange Situation behavior of these "unclassifiable" infants has been undertaken. A first analysis (Main & Solomon, 1986) was based on the Strange Situation behavior of 34 "unclassifiable" infants from our white, middle-class sample. The new analysis and directions for identification presented here are now based upon 80 additional infants, infants whom we have also determined to be unclassifiable (disorganized), and who are largely taken from high-risk and from maltreatment samples. Thus, our findings are no longer confined to the behavior of infants seen in stable, middle-class samples.

Our study of the exact behaviors exhibited by these infants in response to the Ainsworth Strange Situation has shown that those infants who cannot be classified within the traditional A, B, C system do not resemble one another in coherent ways. Specifically, our review of the Strange Situation video-tapes of over 120 unclassifiable infants has failed to date to reveal any patterns of behavior with organized commonalities, that is, new D, E, F, G categories. Rather, what we observe in these infants is any of a diverse array of conflict behaviors indicative of disorganization and disorientation, and probably often indicative of an experience of stress with which they have no means to cope (Main & Hesse, 1990).

In independent analyses of the Adult Attachment Interview, we have found that the parents of these infants have often experienced unresolved, traumatic, attachment-related events – certainly in many cases, loss of an attachment figure through death prior to maturity (Main & Hesse, 1990), and probably other traumas such as physical or sexual abuse involving the attachment figure. There is a strong association between infant disorganized/disoriented attachment status and the parent's lack of resolution of mourning within our

Berkeley sample. Recently, this finding has been replicated within a sample observed in Charlottesville, Virginia (Ainsworth & Eichberg, 1991).

The Adult Attachment Classifications: Secure/Autonomous With Respect to Attachment (B); Dismissing of Attachment (A); Pre-Occupied With Past Attachments (C); Disorganized Through Lack of Resolution of Mourning (D)

Perhaps the most central study in what I have elsewhere (Main et al., 1985) termed the "move to the level of representation" in attachment is the method developed for classificatory analysis of verbatim speech transcripts (Main & Goldwyn, this volume). This system was initially based upon study of transcripts of the Berkeley Adult Attachment Interview (George et al., (1985); this volume), an interview designed to assess the adult's "internal working model" (Bowlby, 1969; Bretherton, 1985) of the "self in relationship to attachment" at the present time. In this interview, the adult is asked specifically to describe her relationships with parents in general terms, then to offer supporting memories, and then to evaluate and interpret memories of attachment-related experiences and their influences. The classification system is not designed to reveal the type of relationship which the adult actually experienced with any particular attachment figure during childhood, but rather to determine the adult's present, attachment-related state of mind. An adult with a history of insecure relationships to parents is, therefore, judged secure in terms of her present state of mind if she can discuss her early experiences with her parents and the probable influences of those experiences coherently, neither idealizing nor exhibiting an excessive present involvement and anger.

When the interview classification system was in its initial stages of development, only three general categories were delineated – *secure/autonomous* with respect to attachment and attachment history; *dismissing of attachment*; and *pre-occupied with previous attachments* –categories corresponding to the secure, insecure-avoidant, and insecure-resistant groups, respectively. Several sub-categories were also developed (interestingly, more adult sub-categories were recognized than corresponding infant sub-categories).

The category system was based upon a development sample of 36 transcripts, and then applied (blind) to the remaining 66 cases. Developing the system involved moving (blind) through each transcript in the development sample, and in each instance using feedback ("correct" or "incorrect" with respect to the infant's attachment classification to that adult) to refine and to further develop the rule system.

This is a slow-moving, but highly profitable method of rule-development, and it was used in the creation of every succeeding system. The method relies philosophically upon the presumption that there will be some attachment-related predictability to behavior in samples (such as the Berkeley sample) in which major life-changes and stresses have not frequently disrupted either child–parent interaction patterns or the child's developing representational models of the relationship. It is important to stress that the application of this method cannot lead empirically to the inflation of actual levels of predictability. An observer who attempts to identify the early attachment organization of any new individual on the basis of provisional rules constructed to describe commonalities observed in the behavior of the several prior individuals assessed, will consistently mis-identify that new individual if either: (a) there is in fact no order, lawfulness, or connection between response to reunion at 1 year and the adult or child assessment under investigation, or if (b) accurate rules have been developed for the first-to-sixth-year equivalencies or adult-to-infant equivalencies across the sample as a whole, but this particular individual fails to fit to pattern. In other words, taking first- to sixth-year predictability as an example, a "hit" will *not* be made if, in fact, the relation between first-year and sixth-year behavior is, in general, chaotic, nor will it be made if this individual belongs to the minority of children in the sample who have changed in attachment organization. "Hits" (matches between adult and infant attachment classifications, or first- and sixth-year classifications) will occur beyond the chance level only if most of the infant behaviors do, in fact, relate systematically to the adult transcripts (or to behaviors 5 years later) in the manner being expressed by the rule system (for example, for 16 among the previous 20 cases). Cases of genuine misfit or instability will necessarily be detected, as they will be represented through the judge's failure to correctly identify the infant attachment pattern.

Of course, once the basic patterns have been identified by the first judge, the system must be tested (blind) with a new judge and upon a new sample. In my view, this method maximizes the likelihood of the discovery of new, attachment-associated patterns.

In determining our adult-to-infant hit-rate, "forced" A, B, C classifications were used for each infant. This was possible because, whenever an infant is determined to be disorganized/disoriented during the Strange Situation, a best-fitting, alternative "Ainsworth" or "A, B, C" classification is still assigned. Including these inherently difficult "D" cases in terms of their best-fitting A, B, or C category, our adult-to-infant-strange-situation hit-rate was 72%. What was particularly impressive even in this first of our studies was our ability to identify the mental organization of parents of insecure-resistant (C) infants as distinct from the mental organization of parents of insecure-avoidant (A) infants. Of the nine adult transcripts in which the adult was judged *pre-occupied with early attachments,* seven had infants who had been judged insecure-resistant with them 5 years previously, and none had infants judged insecure-avoidant. Only 1 out of 26 parents judged *dismissing of attachment* had an infant who had been insecure-resistant. Thus, a highly satisfactory distinction between the mental organization of the parents of A as opposed to C infants had been uncovered.

These results have now been replicated in a Charlottesville sample, in which the adult-to-infant hit-rate was 82% across the three major (A, B, C) categories (Eichberg, doctoral thesis in preparation, 1987). One encouraging advance made in this doctoral thesis is the significant (though low, e.g., 52%) hit-rate obtained for adult-to-infant attachment sub-groups. Thus, the adult as well as the infant classification system provides eight sub-groups of security, and infant sub-categories were predicted at levels well above chance.

In addition, working with the South German (Regensburg) sample being studied by Klaus and Karin Grossmann, Elizabeth Fremmer-Bombik has developed a refined, numerically based method for specifying the differences between adults who are secure/autonomous and adults who are dismissing of attachment (e.g., one variable assessed is the number of memories which involve attachment-related events). Using this refined method, Fremmer-Bombik has also obtained a high (78%) hit-rate for distinguishing mothers of A from mothers of B infants (Grossmann et al., 1988).

Finally, the Adult Attachment Interview has been used in two studies which do not attempt to replicate the original relationships between the adult's attachment classification and the infant's, but rather extend application of the new Adult Attachment Classification System to the prediction of adolescent (Kobak & Sceery, 1988) or mother and toddler (Crowell & Feldman, 1988) behavior in other settings. Using the Block personality Q-sort, Kobak and Sceery (1988) found that adolescents judged Secure/Autonomous in terms of the Adult Attachment Classification System were highly ego-resilient, as determined from independent peer evaluations. This is a particularly encouraging finding because it replicates, at the adolescent level in Charlottesville, a relationship between security of attachment and ego-resilience first uncovered at the kindergarten level by Sroufe (Arend et al., 1979). In addition, Kobak and Sceery (1988) found significant differences between the two groups of insecure adolescents. Adolescents judged dismissing of attachment (the adult "A" classification) in terms of the interview system were described by peers as low on ego-resilience and relatively high on hostility, while adolescents judged pre-occupied by previous attachments (the adult equivalent to the insecure-resistant infant group "C") were viewed instead as anxious. In a recent study, almost identical differences between the social behavior of 5-year-old children who had been insecure-avoidant and insecure-resistant with mother as infants has been uncovered by Sroufe (1983). Thus, whether assessments are made with young children, using the Ainsworth Strange Situation, or are made with young adults, using the Adult Attachment Interview, the Pattern A attachment organization is associated with socially observed hostility, while the Pattern C attachment organization is associated with anxiety.

In Crowell's study, mother's adult attachment classifications predicted both mother's and toddler's behavior in an independently assessed tool-using situation designed by Matas et al. (1978). Again, the behavior of mothers and toddlers in dyads in which mother's transcript had been judged dismissing of attachment differed sharply from those in which the mother had been judged pre-occupied.

Recent work with the Adult Attachment Interview has involved the development of a scale for lack of resolution of mourning of attachment figures lost through death. The two central indications of lack of resolution of mourning are (1) irrational statements or indications of irrational thought processes (e.g., this statement by a highly intelligent professional man: "I still believe my mother died that night because I forgot to pray for her"), and (2) indications that the adult has entered a special state of mind during the discussion of the loss or of the lost figure. Often, this involves some disorientation with respect to the discourse expectancies of the immediate interview context (e.g., "she was young, she was lovely, she was beloved by all who knew her, and yet she was torn from us by that most dreaded of diseases, cancer").

It is the scores derived from this scale, which specifically predict the infant "D" attachment category. Thus, an adult can be both classified as best-fitting at the general "A, B, C" level to the *secure/autonomous* adult attachment category and yet receive a score on the scale for lack of resolution of mourning, which is high enough to predict disorganized/disoriented status for the infant. Such an adult can be readily imagined, given a background of substantially secure relationships to parents, and a family tragedy orphaning the child in circumstances in which there could be self-blame. (The expected infant attachment category in such cases is, of course, D (disorganized/disoriented), with an alternative, "forced" B category.)

To my knowledge, this structured, hour-long interview is the first method of assessment of its type that is tied to a validity measure, which so specifically reflects the speaker's actions outside of the interview context. Thus, *the adult attachment categories not only have face validity but also have been keyed to the adult's behavior as reflected in the infant's security or in any of three types of insecurity of the infant's attachment.*

As anyone who has served as a subject in the interview will attest, spoken responses to the interview questions are almost impossible to control. Hence, the interview will be of assistance not only in helping the clinician or therapist at intake, or as part of an early set of assessments of a patient but also in assessing the course and the success of therapy.

In addition, at the time of this writing, three studies using the interview prior to the birth of the child are underway. If the interview succeeds in predicting infant Strange Situation behavior at 1 year within these studies, clinicians may well be able to assist in the prevention of some potentially detrimental effects of parenting prior to birth.

My own interests in the interview technique at this time involve a deeper attention to its pragmatic and linguistic elements, as well as to the apparent organization of autobiographical memories. The speech of individuals classified as secure/autonomous (who in turn, of course, have infants classified as secure in relationship to them) has a direct, relaxed quality and does not include much that is distancing, dysfluent, or idiosyncratic, in terms of following self-determined rules. The speech of the parents of insecure-avoidant infants involves, not unexpectedly, much distancing (exemplified in the extreme by one parent who referred to "the father" and "the mother"); in addition, in response to the interviewer's search for memories, these parents frequently report a lack of memory for childhood, or, in attempting to respond, move logically from the expectable to the inferred particular, for example, "I *think I probably* went to my mother when I was upset in childhood."

Finally, the memories of the parents of the insecure-resistant infants seem chaotic and unorganized. Often, a flood of memories is presented which does not seem to support any particular generalization regarding experience or the evaluation of experience, nor is the adult, herself, typically able to provide a coherent overview. These parents contrast sharply with the parents of insecure-avoidant infants in that they sometimes claim to remember early childhood especially well. Usage of jargon as substitution for more precise descriptions of early relationships and their effects (e.g., with respect to the likely effects of experience, "I've just got a lot of garbage in my head"; or with respect to why the mother affected the subject as she did, "what was it about her? well, she really pushed my buttons") is not uncommon. In addition, the pre-occupied parents of insecure-resistant infants sometimes show a startling slippage into the present tense in reporting past experiences, and an occasional use of nonsense phrases to complete a sentence (e.g., "So, she just went on and, you know, well, dididididi"). These interviews will, no doubt, provide much new material for the linguist, and, in my view, critical pilot work for the student of memory willing to begin with naturalistic observations of autobiography.

The Parent–Child Discourse Classifications: Fluent (B), Restricted (A), and Dysfluent (D) Discourse

Speech transcripts were made from the 3-minute parent–child reunions which ended the sixth-year assessment procedure. Our intention was to attempt to determine the structure of the relationship between the speakers through the use of words alone. The reunion transcripts were therefore marked for pause and speaker overlap, but devoid of cues to prosody, intonation, or ongoing non-verbal behavior. The transcripts were then given to a psycholinguist, who employed the same system of rule-development described earlier. The judge was familiar with Strange Situation analyses, Adult Attachment analyses, and the behavior of parents of differing classifications during the Clown Session conducted in infancy (Main & Weston, 1981). The judge had not seen these dyads in any context other than the discourse transcripts.

In this phase of our study, too few Group C (insecure-resistant) dyads were available to form a "Group C" discourse classification pattern. Consequently, discourse transcript equivalencies were developed only for dyads in which the infant had been judged secure, insecure-avoidant, or insecure-disorganized/disoriented during infancy. The discourse classifications judged to correspond to these early attachment organizations were identified as *fluent*, *restricted*, and *dysfluent*. In addition, four sub-categories of fluent discourse were developed which paralleled the four sub-categories of secure infant attachment;

and two sub-categories of restricted discourse were developed in parallel to the two sub-categories of insecure-avoidant attachment.

The judge had an overall A, B, D hit-rate to infancy of approximately 80% for both mother–child and father–child dyads (34 mother–child and 32 father–child transcripts). Remarkably, when the seven discourse groups were compared to the corresponding seven infancy groups (A1, A2, B1, B2, B3, B4, and D), 67% of the discourse sub-categories correctly identified the 6-year-old's Strange Situation behavior 5 years earlier (Strage & Main, 1985). Sub-group results comparable to these have not been obtained in any other assessment in our follow-up study, and could be partially due to chance factors. It should be remembered, however, that in comparison to all other of our assessments, discourse classifies the *dyad* rather than the behavior, memories, or drawings of one particular individual. Given that the infant's Strange Situation behavior is a product of dyadic interaction, it may well be that a "dyadic" classification scheme will optimize chances for identifying the organization of the relationship. Indeed, it would be surprising if this were not the case.

Recently, Ulrike Wartner and her colleagues have replicated the association between the child's Strange Situation classification to mother in infancy, and corresponding classifications of parent–child discourse at 6 years of age (Wartner et al., 1994). This replication is particularly impressive, given that the original language of the Regensburg speakers, Bavarian, is not a written language. Hence, a High German translation of the Bavarian speech was first made, before the transcripts were translated a second time for usage by two English speaking judges blind to all other assessments of parent and child.

I see this new, structured approach to the analysis of child–parent discourse as a potentially important influence in the field of discourse studies. While both theoretical and empirical clusterings of qualities of mother–child discourse have been attempted in recent years, these clusters have lacked an anchor in situations external to the dialogue. Thus, investigators have been able to conclude, from rational examinations of clusters of speech acts, that they may well reflect relationships of a particular type. Sources of external validation for these typologies have, however, been lacking. The external validation we now provide is, of course, not more speech in a separate context but a structured relationship observed entirely in terms of non-verbal behavior 5 years earlier.

A study of the discourse transcripts themselves suggests to me that the dyad is active in preserving its own particular form of relationship. This is particularly true in the case of the insecure dyads, whose discourse behavior is the most predictable and the most rule-bound.

Child Family Drawing Classifications: Realistic (B); Invulnerable (A); Vulnerable (C); or Irrational (D)

The system of rule-development described earlier was again used in the classification of children's family drawings. The drawings had been collected as part of a child-examiner "warm-up" period within the Berkeley sixth-year follow-up study. Instructions to the child simply involved (a) asking the child to draw "anything you would like" and then (b) asking the child to draw her family. The set of 36 drawings was then examined, and an attempt was made to determine, on the basis of the overall composition of the drawing (and not at all on the basis of the child's skill), the likely nature of early attachment to the mother.[1] The impression which we gradually gathered with respect to the drawings was that:

(1) some were rational and *realistic* (these were the drawings of children who had been secure with mother in infancy);
(2) some seemed an attempt to portray the family as perfect, highly conformed, cheerful, and *invulnerable* (these were the drawings of children who had been insecure-avoidant with mother in infancy);
(3) some seemed to portray the family either as overwhelming, (e.g., huge), or overwhelmed (e.g., extremely small figures in a corner), alternative configurations which we have termed as *vulnerable* (these were the drawings of children who had been insecure-resistant with mother in infancy); and
(4) some drawings in addition contained *irrational* elements (these were the drawings of children who had been termed insecure-disorganized/disoriented as infants).

Moving blind through the set of drawings while developing the rules for identifying the classifications, the two original judges independently obtained hit-rates of close to 80%. The drawings and the rule system were then given to a third blind judge who had not participated in the development of the system: This judge obtained an overall hit-rate of 76%.

This finding too has been replicated using a South German sample (Wartner et al., 1994). Interestingly, Wartner had found earlier that another well-known system of analysis of children's drawings in terms of "clinical indicators" failed to discriminate the drawings of children who had been secure from the drawings of children who had been insecure in infancy (Wartner, 1987).

Classification of Video-Taped Child Reunion Responses: Secure (B), Insecure-Avoidant (A), Insecure-Resistant (C), and Insecure-Controlling (D)

A judge familiar with the classification of infant Strange Situation behavior patterns examined the video-taped parent–child reunions which ended the sixth-year follow-up study (described earlier). The same process of identification and feedback described earlier was used to develop the rule system for sixth-year "attachment classifications." Children who had been secure with the parent in infancy were relatively simple to identify as *secure* at six, and children who had been avoidant in infancy were also fairly readily identified again as *avoidant*. Children who had been insecure-resistant with the parent in infancy retained noticeable *ambivalence*, together with some exaggerated expressions of dependence. Development of a system of rules for the classification of children who had been disorganized with a given parent in infancy was, however, much more difficult. Rather than exhibiting the conflict behaviors which had led to their "D" Strange Situation classification, most of these children had become *controlling* of the parent through punitive or caregiving behavior. One child seemed insecure while not fitting to any of the above descriptors. Specifically, her behavior toward her father seemed somewhat sexualized. Therefore, we left the system open to include the category, *insecure-unclassified*.

In all, four (A, B, C, D) sixth-year attachment categories were developed, and in addition the open, insecure-unclassified (U) category was utilized. The developed rule system was then given to a judge who was blind to the behavior of the dyads in all other contexts, and was, as well, unfamiliar with categories of infant Strange Situation behavior. This judge found 84% of child–mother reunions predictable from infant attachment classifications to mother, but only 62% of child–father reunions predictable from infant attachment classifications to father.[2]

In a subsequent study at the University of Virginia, Charlottesville, 50 6-year-olds were observed with mother in two similar reunion situations 1 month apart (Main & Cassidy, 1988). Two judges blind to the alternative session assessed the stability of A, B, C, D categories over the 1-month period. The "stability" of A, B, C, D attachment organization over the 1-month period was significant but low (62%), whereas when "D" children were assigned to their best-fitting alternative "A, B, C" categories, stability over the month was high (86%).

The instability of the "D" category over the 1-month period is puzzling, and could be due to a number of factors still to be determined (including a weakness in the classification system, since corrected). However, when each of the 50 children (including the D children) was assigned to an A, B, or C category and sub-category, stability over the month was high even for sub-categories.

Recently, using the South German sample collected by Klaus and Karin Grossmann, Ulrike Wartner has been able to replicate the findings of the Berkeley study. Using the system of sixth-year attachment classification developed in Berkeley and refined in Charlottesville, Wartner has obtained an 84% (A, B, C, D) first-to-sixth-year hit-rate for child–mother dyads (child–father dyads were not included in her study). In addition, the sixth-year system is now receiving support from extensive home observations being made by Solomon, George, and Ivins (1987). They report substantial and expectable associations between the interactions of mothers with their 6-year-olds in the home situation (6 hours of observation) and attachment classifications as determined from the sixth-year reunion procedure. Mothers of 6-year-olds judged secure in terms of the system are described as relatively sensitive and accepting toward the child in the home situation, while mothers of children judged insecure-avoidant at six are described as relatively rejecting and avoidant of physical contact.

Summary

The discoveries briefly reviewed above present a new level of evidence regarding the degree of structure, coherence, and predictability in behavior. Four major attachment organizations, as classified in infancy, are now shown capable of predicting the quality of children's drawings, discourse, and expressive behavior toward the parent at six. In addition, the prediction of these same infant attachment organizations from the parents' spoken representations and evaluations of their own attachment histories suggests an entirely new specificity of linkage between the mind of one person and the behavior of another. The findings show that the preservation of attachment relationships of particular types – as well as the representational models of those relationships – involves the participation of cognitive mechanisms which include not only language usage, but also perception, and, in all probability, the organization of autobiographical memory.

These methods provide opportunities for research not only in the area of attachment but also in such fields as linguistics, cognition, memory, and perception. In addition, they create new bases for clinical diagnosis and intervention. Figures 1.1–1.4 provide a brief summary of the methods described above. The reader may wish to review these figures to gain a clearer overall conceptualization of the contents of this volume before a detailed examination of the methods themselves is undertaken.

Notes

1 I believe it is possible that the early organization of attachment to the father as well as the mother might be reflected in these family drawings. In this series of assessments of representational models of attachment, however, the organization of the relationship to the mother was most easy to determine. (For a discussion of why this may be so, see Main et al., 1985).

2 The low, though still significant, infancy-to-sixth-year hit-rate for fathers has still to be explained. Since father–child discourse was predicted from infant attachment to father as successfully as mother–child discourse, it is too early to assume that the father–child relationship is unstable. It may be, however, that it is more accurately reflected in discourse than in non-verbal behavior, a hypothesis supported by several previously secure children who physically avoided or else disobeyed the father at six, while engaging in fluent discourse.

2 Procedures for Identifying Infants as Disorganized/ Disoriented During the Ainsworth Strange Situation

Mary Main and Judith Solomon

This chapter is reprinted in part from: M. Greenberg, D. Cichetti, & M. Cummings, *Attachment in the Preschool Years*. Chicago: University of Chicago Press, 1990 (Greenberg et al., 1990). This chapter describes a method for identifying particular forms of infant conflict behavior – which we have termed "disorganized and/or disoriented" behaviors – within the Ainsworth Strange Situation. We have reason to believe (Wartner, 1987) that the method will work equally well to identify these behaviors in settings other than the Ainsworth Strange Situation, that is, in a mildly stressful infant–parent–stranger observation (the Clown Session designed by Main & Weston (1981)). Since, however, the method is likely to be applied by most investigators to observations of parent and infant made within the Strange Situation, we begin the chapter with a brief description of Ainsworth's system. We move then to tracing the history of the development of our method. Finally, we present directions for determining that an individual infant is disorganized/disoriented.

The Ainsworth Strange Situation. The Ainsworth Strange Situation is a brief, laboratory-based observation of the infant's response to two separations from, and reunions with, the parent (Ainsworth et al., 1978). Infant responses to this situation are classified in one of three patterns: secure (the infant greets the parent positively upon reunion, identified as "group B" behavior); insecure-avoidant (the infant actively avoids the parent upon reunion, identified as "group A" behavior); or insecure-resistant (the infant shows mild to obvious resistance to the parent, and an inability to be settled, identified as "group C" behavior). Individual differences in infant response to a particular parent in this situation are thought to reflect corresponding differences in the history of interaction which the infant has experienced with that parent, and to predict important differences in later functioning (Bretherton, 1985).

Investigators working with middle-class parent–infant dyads have typically placed each infant seen in the Strange Situation in one of these three major "attachment classifications," despite the difficulties presented by the occasional infant whose behavior does not precisely fit to a category. In a first publication, however (Main & Solomon, 1986), we described the Strange Situation behavior of 55 infants whose response to separation and reunion had failed to meet either Group A, Group B, or Group C classification criteria

DOI: 10.4324/9781003569978-2

as described by Ainsworth and her colleagues (Ainsworth et al., 1978). Given that the three original A, B, C attachment categories had been discovered on the basis of the response variation found among only 23 infant–mother dyads, we expected that in a sample of unclassifiable infants this large, a number of different, coherent, and distinct, that is, "D," "E," "F," and "G" responses (categories) might be uncovered.

The central discovery which we reported in our first paper was the absence of clear new categories of infant Strange Situation behavior within this sample (Main & Solomon, 1986). Infants who could not be classified within the present, "A, B, C" system did not appear to us to resemble one another in Strange Situation behavior in coherent, organized ways. What these infants shared in common other than their failure to be classifiable within the present system was bouts or sequences of behavior which seemed to observers to lack a readily observable and coherent goal, intention, or explanation. The term we selected to describe these diverse behavior patterns was "disorganized and/or disoriented." In some infants, behavior could be seen as disorganized only when it was considered at an abstract level, as a disorganized (disordered) sequencing of otherwise well-organized behavior patterns – for example, strong avoidance of the parent directly succeeding strong proximity-seeking, termed by us "disordering of expected temporal sequences." In other infants, there were distinct episodes in which the infant showed disorganization in behavior (e.g., approaching with head averted) or in which the infant seemed disoriented (stilling or freezing of movement for 30 seconds with a dazed expression). We described the behavior of these "D" (disorganized/disoriented) infants as including one or more of the following features: *disordering of expected temporal sequences; simultaneous display of contradictory behavior patterns; incomplete or undirected movements and expressions, including stereotypies; direct indices of confusion and apprehension;* and *behavioral stilling*. Different indices of disorganization and disorientation appeared in different infants.

The primary intention of this chapter is, of course, to provide a clear enough description of disorganization and disorientation in infant Strange Situation behavior that the reader can identify the pattern in other samples. In addition, however, the reader may wish to know (a) whether we have evidence that this type of Strange Situation behavior could be a function of neurological or other difficulties experienced by the infant as an individual rather than as a function of a particular relationship; (b) whether this category could be associated with any particular experience the infant or parent may have undergone; and (c) whether, like the traditional A, B, and C Strange Situation categories, this new category of Strange Situation behavior has distinct sequelae in later childhood. In earlier and separate papers, we have established the following regarding the "D" attachment category:

1. "D" attachment status is independent across caregivers. In view of the nature of the behaviors being exhibited by these infants, it seemed particularly relevant to address the issue of whether disorganized/disoriented

behavior could be simply a function of neurological or other difficulties being experienced by the infant at a particular point in time, and having little to do with the relational issues which concern most research in attachment. In our earlier paper (Main & Solomon, 1986), we presented data from the Berkeley Social Development Project in which each infant was seen with both parents, one at 12, the other at 18 months of infant age. Of the 34 Strange Situations judged "D" within this sample, only three involved the same infant. Out of the 34 infants, 31 were disorganized only in the presence of one parent. Comparable evidence for independence of "unclassifiable" attachment status across caregivers was presented in a doctoral thesis completed by Krentz (1982), reviewed in Main and Solomon, (1986).[1] These findings suggest that D attachment status might have its origin in the history of the infant's interaction with the parent.

2. We do not have an observational base for determining the parent–infant interaction patterns in dyads in which the infant is classified D within the Strange Situation. However, we have strong evidence that the parents of "D" infants differ in their own attachment-related experiences from other parents. We find that infant "D" attachment status is strongly associated with the parent's loss of a parent through death prior to completion of high school, and that it is even more strongly associated with lack of resolution of mourning of attachment figures lost through death at any age period (Main, 1983; Main & Hesse, this volume). There is also some evidence to suggest that it may be associated with other major attachment-related traumas experienced by the parent, such as sexual or physical abuse.
3. Infants who are categorized "D" with a particular parent in infancy are distinguishable from other children for their reunion behavior toward that parent 5 years later: many of these previously disorganized children show a new form of organization in relationship to the parent (controlling or role-reversing). These findings are based upon observation of the Berkeley Social Development Project children in a video-taped sixth-year reunion procedure with each parent (Main & Cassidy, 1988). Reunion assessments were conducted by individuals who were blind to infant attachment status. A majority of the children who had been categorized D with the parent in infancy were controlling of the parent (either controlling-punitive or controlling-caregiving) as 6-year-olds. In addition, family drawings of children who had been categorized D as infants were distinguishable from the drawings of A, B, and C infants (Kaplan & Main, 1986). (Still other sequelae seen at 6 years of age are described in Main et al. (1985)).

To date, we have reviewed the (video-taped) Strange Situation behavior of a total of 120 video-tapes of infants whom we judged to be disorganized/disoriented in terms of their Strange Situation behavior. Whereas 34/55 "D" infants in our earlier report came from our stable, upper-middle-class sample, most of the new "D" infants studied for the purposes of this chapter come from lower-class families. In total, we have now reviewed 37 video-tapes of "D" infants from high-risk samples, and 20 of infants from abusing and/or neglecting families. Our analysis of Strange-Situation video-tapes of these infants indicates that the "D" classification criteria which identify these "not A, B, or C" infants in normal samples serve equally well to identify "not A, B, or C" infants from maltreatment, high-risk and poverty samples.

The purpose of this chapter is to formally present a set of indices of disorganization and disorientation in Strange Situation behavior which will permit the identification of "D" infants by other workers. We (a) discuss the theoretical considerations which influenced our development of a new classification and the process by which we developed and obtained reliability for the classification criteria to be presented; (b) present the classification criteria; and (c) discuss the issue of category demarcation.

Theoretical Considerations and Steps Taken in the Development of the Disorganized/Disoriented Strange Situation Category

The new "D" category of infant Strange Situation behavior has been developed over a period of several years. In this section, we review what we now see as the critical steps which we took in the development of this new category. We describe this process in some detail because we believe that beyond its immediate interest as documentation of our methods, it illustrates one approach to the more general problems involved in the modification of an existing, and largely successful, classification system.

Questions regarding the basis upon which additional classifications should be developed are relatively new to students of attachment, but have long been confronted in other areas of psychology and in other disciplines. We feel it will be helpful to other workers in this field, now in a new phase of expansion and discovery, to highlight theoretical issues and aspects of the classificatory process which have guided our own work.

Theoretical issues in the modification of classification systems

We have found it helpful to draw upon evolutionary biology, a science with a long history of grappling with the development and modification of classificatory systems. A central question in biological systematics has been the source of classification, that is, whether the organism's phylogenetic history exclusively, or its appearance exclusively, or some combination of history and appearance should be used to develop new categories. Our own position with respect to behavioral classification parallels that of Mayr (1976) with respect to species classifications. We are interested at once in behavioral appearance (infant Strange Situation behavior) and in the infant's interactional history. Behavioral appearance (i.e., specific behaviors which characterize disorganized/disoriented infants) is not of interest in itself, but for its ability to reveal the ways in which individually differing histories of experience act to shape representational and behavioral processes. Interactional history, of itself, is also not of interest unless we can arrive at an understanding of its consequences for mental and behavioral organization.

A second major issue in systematics concerns the meaning of classification once determined. Here the central question is whether classifications are "created" and artifactual entities, reflecting arbitrary cuts in continuous variables (the nominalist position), or whether classifications reflect an underlying natural order (the realist position). The nominalist approach to Strange Situation classification would not distinguish or differentially weigh indices of insecurity with respect to potential underlying differences in function (i.e., attachment strategy) or with respect to developmental history.

Our own position with respect to classification is that of the realist. The several attachment classifications recognized to date are assumed to represent meaningful rather than arbitrary differences in ontology. That is, while the boundaries and definitions of categories may be improved upon, they represent systematic differences in attachment strategy stemming from significant variations in interactional history.

Our realist position with respect to behavior classification has permitted our discovery of the disorganized/disoriented attachment patterns. We began with attention to behavior form and moved from this to discoveries regarding a particular experiential history. We had no knowledge of infant attachment history when we set aside infants who seemed to fail to fit any of the original classificatory criteria. But this exacting attention to "appearance" led us to the later discovery of corresponding differences in "history," that is, to the discovery of the effects of the parent's early loss of an attachment figure (Main & Hesse, this volume). In the future, recognition of other distinctions in the parent's or infant's history may lead us to search for further corresponding differences in form, while increasing recognition of differences in behavioral form may lead to further discoveries regarding differences in history.

Development of the disorganized/disoriented Strange Situation category depended upon our initial recognition that some infants cannot be classified within the A, B, C system, a recognition which led to the use of an "unclassifiable" category (Main & Weston, 1981). Here, we review what we now see as the critical steps which we took in the development of this new category.

1. We noted that the Strange Situation behavior of some infants could not be described within the A, B, C classification system (Main & Weston, 1981). Infants who could not be classified as A, B, or C within our white, middle-class Berkeley sample were set apart from other infants as early as 1977, but without further specification as to direct indices of special status. Thus, our earlier work was based entirely upon the failure of the Strange Situation behavior of individual infants to fit to classification descriptors (Ainsworth et al., 1978).

During the initial period in which infants in our laboratory were set aside as "unclassifiable," we were largely noting inconsistencies and incoherencies in "A," "B," or "C" behavior during the Strange Situation. This in effect amounts to inconsistencies in what can broadly be termed attachment strategies.

In general, the attachment behavioral system is organized to maintain varying degrees of proximity between infant and parent, and to intensify proximity or contact between infant and parent in situations of threat or alarm (Bowlby, 1969). Because the conditions facing the *parent* may be different at different times (or in different cultural or ecological contexts), however, the system can be readily understood to permit organized variations in infant behavior in response to coherent variations in the behavior of the parent (Main, 1981; Hinde, 1982). Under some ecological or cultural ("Group A") conditions, it will be to the parent's advantage to stress early independence for the infant, resulting in relative rejection of some forms of attachment behavior; under other ecological or cultural ("Group C") conditions, the parent may emphasize infant dependence. Shifts in parental and infant strategy over quite brief periods are not unexpectable; however, within a particular period, both parental and infant behavior are expected to be relatively well-organized.

At an abstract level, the infant attachment organization corresponding to the parent's caregiving strategies can be described quite briefly as a set of attachment-related "instructions" or "strategies" (Main & Solomon, 1986; see also the discussion of infant attachment organization in Sroufe & Waters, 1977). We see the following sets of "strategies" as describing much of the Strange Situation behavior of infants who are classifiable within one of these three categories:

Secure – use the parent as a secure base for exploration while present; show attachment behavior upon separation; use parent as a secure base again upon reunion (Ainsworth et al., 1978).

Avoidant – divert attention from attachment-eliciting cues of any kind (situational or interpersonal) and instead attend to the environment.

Resistant/ambivalent[2] – heighten responsiveness to attachment-eliciting cues, and exaggerate emotionality, particularly fear and anger (also described as heightened dependence, see Trivers, 1974; Main, 1981).

Many of the Ainsworth classification instructions for the A, B, and C categories can be understood as the natural consequence of an infant using these strategies. Given this understanding of the A, B, and C attachment patterns as representing organized attachment strategies (see Sroufe & Waters, 1977), it becomes especially understandable that we had judged as disorganized or as unclassifiable:

(1) potential "group A" infants who were greatly distressed by each separation from the parent, though avoidant on reunions, and thus seemed unable to maintain a "strategy" of diverting attention from attachment;

(2) potential "group B" infants who immediately followed strong proximity-seeking with avoidance; responded to reunion with the parent with an apprehensive expression; or sat or stood immobilized or frozen for substantial periods during reunion rather than either continuing to seek engagement with the parent or returning to play; and

(3) potential "Group C" infants[2] who failed to cry upon separation and/or alternately exhibited distress and moderate to strong avoidance, thus violating the expectancy of a consistent heightening of attachment behavior.

Although (in the following section) we present a list of direct indices of disorganization and disorientation during the Strange Situation, it is also important to keep in mind the original, sheerly exclusion ("not A, B, or C") criteria which identified the same set of infants as being disorganized in terms of failure to adhere to any of the three major attachment strategies.

2. *We decided to review the 36 "unclassifiable" Berkeley Strange Situation video-tapes to determine specifics of their Strange Situation behavior.* The central question was: What kinds of behavioral indices should be relied upon as the basis for additional classifications? One possibility (as noted earlier) was to confine ourselves to attempting to identify new combinations of the several individual scores assigned to infants when the video-tapes are first reviewed. These scores often include records of crying by the infant during the entire Strange Situation, and always include scores assigned to the infant in terms of the four interactive scoring systems devised by Ainsworth, that is, proximity-seeking, proximity-avoiding, contact-maintaining, and contact-resisting during each reunion (Ainsworth et al., 1978). Infants who showed combinations of these behaviors not consonant with the A, B, and C classifications could have then been assigned to new classifications.

This method seemed inadequate; however, since many of the behaviors which we had observed and which had led to "unclassifiable" infant attachment status were not contributors to any of the interactive scoring systems. One infant, for example, met the classification criteria for Group B except for a look of apprehension which appeared briefly and immediately upon each reunion and was accompanied by a fearful expression and by placing her hand over her mouth. Neither fearful expressions nor the hand-to-mouth gesture enters into the avoidance or resistance scoring systems, yet these are gestures, which seem clearly inconsonant with security.

Similarly, another infant met the criteria for Group C except for a long period of "freezing" movement (stilling) during each reunion episode. She had high resistance scores and indeed all interactive and crying scores were consonant with the C classification. Stilling – the behavior pattern which had led us to decide not to classify this infant – was not recorded through any of the original scoring systems.

In sum, the behaviors, which had led us to the conclusion that a given infant was unclassifiable, were not recorded as contributors to any of the four interactive scoring systems. In addition, these behaviors were often exhibited by infants whose scores were well matched to those described by Ainsworth as representative for a particular attachment classification, for example, high scores for avoidance and low or zero scores for all other variables in an unclassifiable infant assigned to A1 as a classification. The behavior which had led us to draw any given infant out of the A, B, C classification system could only be identified by a new, direct study of the Strange Situation video-tapes.

3. *We discovered that almost all (34/36) of the "unclassifiable" Berkeley infants showed inexplicable, irrational, odd or conflicted patterns of behavior during the Strange Situation.* Many investigators, including ourselves, expected that a thorough examination of the Strange Situation behavior of infants who could not be classified within the present system would yield a set of several new attachment classifications, for example, D, E, and F attachment classifications. Two of the 36 infants were so casually avoidant that the judges had questioned whether they were attached to the parent with whom they were seen in the Strange Situation (the father). Among the remaining 34 infants, however, no two appeared to resemble one another in Strange Situation behavior sufficiently to warrant the creation of a new category of organized Strange Situation response. Rather, these infants showed a diverse set of inexplicable, unexpectable behavior patterns, some violating temporal expectancies (e.g., crying at the door for the parent, then moving away in strong avoidance immediately upon reunion), some seeming simply disorganized or contradictory (approaching with head averted), some featuring stereotypies (rocking violently on knees and hands), and some suggesting the mutual inhibition of systems in conflict ("freezing" or stilling in movement for long periods). The very lack of organization implicit in this array of diverse behavioral characters mitigated against the conclusion that we had discovered new "patterns of organization" (cf. Ainsworth et al., 1978; Sroufe & Waters, 1977).

4. *We were unable to find a single thematic heading which could describe this set of "inexplicable, irrational, odd or conflicted" behaviors sufficiently to permit recognition of new instances by ourselves and by other workers: No term was considered completely satisfactory – however, "disorganized and/or disoriented" was selected.* The most impressive common theme in the diverse list of "inexplicable, irrational, odd or conflicted" behavior patterns observed in unclassified infants was the simple lack of a clear immediate goal, purpose, or explanation discernible by the observer. Selecting a final descriptive heading for this diverse array of behaviors was, however, difficult. Many of the behaviors could be seen as the outcomes of conflict ("conflict behaviors"). However, "conflict behavior" did not seem a useful heading. Depending upon point of view, the careful observer can see a broad range of infant behaviors as conflict behavior. This term is particularly easy to apply when we consider the Strange Situation behavior of infants in the insecure Ainsworth categories. For example, diverting attention to a toy at the moment of reunion with the parent can be seen as conflict behavior (termed displacement behavior in ethology) as can repeatedly clinging to the parent then pushing away (termed alternation). Thus, "conflict behavior" seemed too broad a category.

The most striking theme running through the list of recorded behaviors was that of *disorganization*. This is a subjective term, intentionally applied only to the infant's overt behavior (and not its mental state), and taking certain expectancies regarding infant behavioral organization and infant intentionality for granted. However, it is easily applied by most observers. For example, contradictory movements, as, approaching parent but with head averted, or at a more abstract level, violations of expected temporal sequences (as, full bright approach to parent followed by sudden avoidance) are readily identified by observers as some kind of disorganization. The term *disorientation* was also needed, because immobilized, dazed behavior, and the assumption of depressed postures, are not literally disorganized but rather seem to signal a lack of orientation to the present environment (for example, episodes of "stilling," of "freezing," or of "depressed affect" in which the infant seems to take no account of the immediate environment). While a review of the actual behaviors observed (Table 2.1) shows that no single title is fully satisfactory, "disorganized/disoriented" seemed reasonably descriptive.

Table 2.1 Direct indices of confusion, disorganization, or disorientation

DIRECT INDICES OF DISORGANIZATION AND DISORIENTATION

A Guide for the Classification of Infants 12–18 Months' Old Behavior Observed with Parent Present

I. DISORDERING OF EXPECTED TEMPORAL SEQUENCES

* Strong proximity-seeking and bright, full greeting upon reunion, followed immediately by moving toward wall or into center of room and stilling with a "dazed" expression.
* Infant is extremely distressed by separation from parent, and cries or calls for parent at the door even when stranger is present: Immediately upon reunion, however, the infant shows strong avoidance.
* Infant calm and undistressed during both separations, but shows distressed, angry, ambivalent behavior upon reunions.
* After a substantial period of settling by the parent and after return to play, sudden out-of-context crying or displays of distressed anger without rationale.
* In the middle of a display of anger and distress, the infant suddenly moves away from and avoids the parent without rationale.
* After strong proximity-seeking and a bright, full greeting, the infant suddenly becomes avoidant.
* Other.

II. SIMULTANEOUS DISPLAY OF CONTRADICTORY BEHAVIOR PATTERNS

* Movements of approach are repeatedly accompanied by movements of avoidance such as the following:

  infant approaches parent with head sharply averted
  infant approaches parent by backing toward parent
  infant reaches arms up for parent with head sharply averted, or with head down

* Distress, clinging, or resistance is accompanied by simultaneous marked avoidance for substantial periods, as:

  infant moves into corner or behind item of furniture while angrily, openly refusing or resisting parent.

* Avoidance of parent, shown in absence of response, silence, or averted head/gaze, is accompanied by distress/anger indices, as:

  infant silently averts head and body away from parent who is offering or attempting pick-up but makes stiff, angry kicking movements and hits hands on floor.

(*Continued*)

Table 1.2 (Continued)

* While held by or holding onto parent, infant shows avoidance of parent:
  infant sits on lap for extended period with averted gaze, ignoring parent's overtures.
  infant holds arms and legs away from parent while permitting self to be held ("starfish" posture).
  infant clings to parent for substantial period while sharply averting gaze, arching away, or averting head from parent.
* Infant impassively strikes, pushes, or pulls against parent's face, eyes, or neck while smiling or in good mood.
* Infant smiles toward parent while looking fearful. For example, infant shows immediate broad "toothy" smile at parent's entrance, but the smile has strong "fear" elements, as, mouth corners tensed, back and down, rigid or frozen eyes.
* Infant approaches parent while simultaneously creating a pathway which avoids and moves away from parent (circling or parabolic pathway).
* Other.

III. **INCOMPLETE, UNDIRECTED, AND INTERRUPTED MOVEMENTS AND EXPRESSIONS**

* *Extensive or intense expressions of distress accompanied by moves away from parent, as infant appears frightened of stranger in parent's presence, moves and leans forehead on wall.*
* Extensive crying in parent's presence without any move toward or look toward the parent.
* Any marked failure to move toward the parent when path is not blocked and infant is clearly distressed or frightened.
* Expression of strong fear or distress regarding an object while staring at it, without withdrawing from it.
* *Exceptionally slow, limp, "underwater" movements of striking at, pushing at, or pulling at the parent's face, eyes, or neck (aggressive intent almost indiscernible).*
* Exceptionally slow, limp "underwater" movements of approach.
* Movements to touch parent are contradicted, that is, infant moves hand toward parent and withdraws hand before touching parent, without rationale.
* Infant interrupts approach to parent on reunion with a bout of resistant behavior, directed away from the parent, and then continues approach.
* Infant begins strong approach upon reunion but interrupts approach briefly to look away and strike hand on floor with angry sounds, then completes full approach.
* Repeated, hesitant, stop–start approach movements (or reach movements) toward parent, giving impression of timidity, apprehension, or indecision.
* Other.

IV. **STEREOTYPIES, ASYMMETRICAL MOVEMENTS, MIS-TIMED MOVEMENTS, AND ANOMALOUS POSTURES**

* *Asymmetries of movement on approach (asymmetrical creeping, heavy or fast on one side only), with or without sudden, unpredictable changes of direction.*
* Asymmetries of facial expression directly upon the appearance of the parent, for example, an extremely swift "tic" which lifts only the left side of the facial musculature.
* Repeated assumption of asymmetries of posture, such as, head-cocking.

(Continued)

Table 1.2 (Continued)

* Stereotypies shown in parent's presence. Rocking, ear-pulling, hair-twisting, and any other rhythmical, repeated movements without visible function. *Pathognomic if marked and repeated while infant is being held by parent.* (Do not include rubbing eyes while in arms, if infant has been crying. Do not include "stereotypies" which make sense in the immediate context, as rubbing eyes in a tired infant).
* Repeated assumption of anomalous, uninterpretable posture. This posture may be stereotyped for a particular baby, as, closing eyes and holding hands forward at shoulder height for several seconds during each reunion.
* Extremely stiff movements and tension in postures, marked in presence of parent but absent during separations.
* Mis-timed movements. Sudden, unpredictable bouts of activity or movement which seem to lack normal preparation time for initiation, and/or which have a jerky, automaton-like (unmonitored) quality. For example, a sudden extreme burst of jerky arm and leg activity in an infant who had been sitting tense and immobilized a second prior.
* Other.

V. **FREEZING, STILLING, SLOW MOVEMENTS AND DEPRESSED AFFECT**

* "Freezing" of apparent intended movement in transit, or interruption of movement, in posture which consequently involves active resistance to gravity. For example, infant sits or stands for 10 seconds with arms held out waist-high and to sides. *Pathognomic if interruptive to a bout of distress or resistance, or if accompanied by "trancelike" facial expression. Pathognomic if lasts more than 20 seconds.* (Do not include first 20 seconds of reunion if infant is being held by parent and has been crying.)
* Marking stilling (stoppage of all natural movement, but infant in easy or "resting" posture). *Pathognomic if lasts more than 15 seconds when held by the parent, or if there are several shorter episodes while held by parent:* However, the first 30 *seconds* after reunion are excluded if the infant has been crying.
  Pathognomic if lasts more than 30 seconds even when infant is not held by the parent.
* *Infant rises or begins approach to parent immediately upon reunion, but falls prone in "depressed" (huddled) posture.*
* *Assuming prone, "depressed" posture for more than 10 seconds at any point in presence of parent, so long as infant is not ill or exhausted.*
* Marked lethargy to movements, impassive, dulled facial expression, and other indices of depressed affect.
* Stilling accompanied by tense, smooth closing of lids.
* Other.

VI. **DIRECT INDICES OF APPREHENSION REGARDING PARENT**[5]

* *Any immediate expression of fear or apprehension directly upon return of parent, or when parent calls or approaches, as:*

  jerking back, with fearful expression.
  anxious over-bright smile or grin with "fear" elements, as, mouth corners drawn back and down.

(*Continued*)

Table 1.2 (Continued)

defensive posture (head drawn into neck, leaning away from parent) with fearful expression.

flinging hands about, over, or in front of face, or over mouth, with fearful expression.

dashing away from the door/parent immediately upon reunion, with hunched or tucked head and shoulders.

* Moving behind chair or behind furniture, out of reach or out of sight of parent without rationale of pursuit of a toy or vigorous exploration *(pathognomic if occurs immediately upon reunion).*
* Following a hesitant or careful approach to the parent with a rapid, tense "away" movement.
* Offering objects to the parent with tense arm and over an unusual distance, as though avoiding parental "reach" space.
* Raising or tensing shoulders when approaching or in contact with parent.
* Highly vigilant posture or appearance when in presence of parent. Movements or posture tense, infant gives impression of being hyper-alert to parent even or especially when parent positioned behind her.
* Assuming defensive stance or posture while looking at parent.
* Other.

VII. **DIRECT INDICES OF DISORGANIZATION OR DISORIENTATION**

* *"Greeting"* stranger *brightly, or approaching stranger with raised* arms immediately as parent enters.
* *Flinging hands over,* about, or in front of face directly upon return of the parent, and in clear response to return of the parent.
* Any clear indices of confusion and disorganization in first moment of reunion with the parent.
* Raising hand or hands to mouth directly upon the return of the parent, as though confused, puzzled, wary, or indecisive. (Do *not include* thumb- or finger-sucking, putting objects in mouth or removing objects from mouth). *Pathognomic if clearly confused/wary.*
* Confused or confusing sequences of very rapid changes of affect in first few seconds of reunion with parent, as, rapid movement of withdrawal accompanied by confused cry-laugh. (Pathognomic feature if marked).
* Pursue parent, protesting departure, and then smile immediately at back of departing parent or at closed door.
* Cry at stranger's leave-taking, and/or rapidly pursue stranger to door as though protesting or pursuing departing parent.
* Disoriented facial expression. Sudden "blind" look to eyes, where infant has previously used eyes normally.
* Fall while approaching parent (exclude tripping over toys). Fall in response to parent reaching for infant. *Fall to floor at hearing parent call from outside of door.*
* Disorganized wandering, especially when accompanied by disoriented expression; overt absence of purpose.
* Other.

Footnote. We have italicized behavior patterns which are pathognomic for assignment to the "D" category, that is, behaviors which immediately and in themselves serve to identify the infant as disorganized/disoriented.

5. *We reviewed these 34 tapes again and constructed a list of the exact behavior patterns which seemed disorganized and/or disoriented.* We reviewed each of the 34 Strange Situation video-tapes and constructed a list of behaviors which seemed to us disorganized/disoriented. We described the disorganized or disoriented behavior in some detail, for example, "infant sits without moving for 35 seconds with hand on mother's knee, looking out and ahead with head turned out away from mother," together with its timing, for example, "beginning of first reunion." Narrative descriptions of the disorganized, disoriented, or otherwise inexplicable behaviors of each infant were recorded.

Once we had completed the analysis of infant (12 or 18 month) Strange Situation behavior in the presence of a given parent (mother or father) for the Berkeley sample, we found 34/268 dyads (12.7%) to be disorganized/disoriented, while 2 were simply left unclassified (were neither classifiable nor disorganized). Of the 34 disorganized cases, the majority (21, or 62%) were judged "secure" in terms of traditional classifications, 8 (23%) were judged "insecure-ambivalent/resistant" in terms of traditional classifications, and 5 (15%) were alternately "insecure-avoidant."

6. *We studied the descriptive record of disorganized/disoriented behaviors seen in these infants with the aim of developing a set of more abstract or thematic headings under which the particular behaviors can be organized.* As noted earlier, the 34 "D" infants were more dissimilar than similar in terms of the exact "D" behavior exhibited. For this reason, no list of exact behaviors could be provided except as behavior examples, and these alone would not enable other researchers to recognize new instances of such behavior. However, study of the list of behaviors exhibited permitted us to identify higher-order themes (e.g., "disordering of expected temporal sequences") which identified the behaviors or behavior sequences which we were seeing, but on a more abstract level. For example, "cries and calls for mother at door, then suddenly becomes avoidant as door opens," "bright, full greeting followed by avoidance," "sudden distressed crying following a casual greeting and return to play" were now ordered under the thematic heading, "disordering of expected temporal sequences."[3] This list of thematically oriented indices of disorganization and disorientation in behavior was organized into a table, "Directions for Identifying Indices of Disorganization and Disorientation." The final version of this table is included as Table 2.1.

7. *We were now several steps from the original classifiable/unclassifiable distinction made within the Berkeley sample.* We now used our *list of thematic headings and behavior examples in reviewing a set of 60* "classifiable" *(A, B, C) infants from the same sample. Our aim was to determine whether these classifiable infants in fact showed the same set of behaviors.* We had originally identified "unclassifiable" infants within the Berkeley sample simply on the basis of their failure to fit to an A, B, or C attachment category. Although we had already established that every infant who had originally been left unclassified either showed one of these indices strongly, or exhibited several of these indices, the possibility remained open that these specific

indices had also been shown by infants earlier determined to be classifiable. In other words, disorganized/disoriented behavior might not have actually been related to the original failure of the infant to meet the Ainsworth classification criteria.

Reviewing Strange Situation tapes of classified (classifiable) infants to determine whether they too showed substantial indices of disorganization and/or disorientation was therefore an important step in the development of the category. Although 7 of the 60 infants came near to "D" attachment status using these identifiers (Main & Solomon, 1986), none matched to the infants previously considered unclassifiable (now, "D") in intensity or timing of these indices. Thus, these indices seemed as expected to distinguish these infants as a separate category.

8. *Are the written "D" classification criteria precise enough to permit us to establish inter-judge reliability (a) in collaboration with an investigator in another laboratory and (b) using Strange Situation video-tapes from a high-risk rather than a middle-class sample?* We forwarded our tables of indices of disorganization and disorientation to a laboratory working with a large, high-risk sample of infants and mothers. Whereas the D system had been developed entirely on the basis of our stable, upper middle-class sample, it would need to be successfully applied to a broad range of samples. We did not provide the second laboratory with video-tapes of "D" infants in our own laboratory, but only with our written descriptions and directions (expertise in the analysis of Strange Situation behavior had already been established for this laboratory). The new judges first re-scored their Strange Situation tapes to include the "D" category, and then forwarded an assortment of tapes including a high proportion of "D" infants to our laboratory. While this work in still in progress, over the first cases, high inter-judge agreement has been obtained for all categories, including the "D" category (Spieker & Booth, 1985).[4] In addition, the D directions successfully captured all infants originally identified as "A–C" within this second sample.

9. *We studied Strange Situation video-tapes loaned to us by investigators working with poverty, high-risk, and/or maltreatment samples in order to broaden our base of examples of disorganized/disoriented behavior, and further clarify our classification criteria.* This chapter is based upon our study of 120 Strange Situation video-tapes in which we have determined that a given infant is disorganized/disoriented. The great majority of these tapes have been loaned to us by other investigators who have been working with these further samples. The group is now fairly evenly divided between infants from middle-class homes and infants from poverty and in many cases welfare families. It includes approximately 20 infants from maltreating families.

Indices of Disorganization and Disorientation

Table 2.1 represents an attempt to order examples of the various types of disorganization and disorientation in behavior seen in the Strange Situation under seven thematic headings. The headings are selected for heuristic purposes: As the reader will note, some patterns of behavior could have been placed under several headings, for example, a fearful smile could be described as "simultaneous exhibition of contradictory behavior patterns" as well as a "direct index of apprehension." We discuss each of these briefly, offering some behavior examples taken from the infants in our own sample who were previously termed "unclassified," and some from video-tapes loaned to us by other investigators.

Disordering of expected temporal sequences. The most striking disordering of expected temporal sequences appeared with respect to avoidance. When an infant ignores and physically avoids the parent throughout the Strange Situation, the infant is classified as avoidant (Ainsworth et al., 1978). When the infant ignores and physically avoids the parent through much of the first reunion episode, then following a second separation seeks proximity, the infant is placed in a mildly avoidant sub-category of "secure" infants. In either case, avoidance is seen as an "organized shift of attention" (Main & Weston, 1982) away from the parent which occurs during and directly following separation. Both an increase in stress (a second separation) and an assurance of continued parental proximity may lead to the replacement of avoidance with proximity-seeking.

Given this usual form of temporal organization, avoidance can be understood as "reserve." Adults not infrequently behave in a reserved manner following long separations, or when uncertain, angry, or apprehensive regarding the current status of a relationship. This reserve may "melt" with time or with assurances from the partner, or in contrast, it may "break down" if the relationship is further threatened (if, for example, the partner threatens to leave again). There is nothing innately disorganized in this usage of avoidance or reserve.

Consider now, in contrast, the temporal organization of avoidance described in Table 2.1. Rather than avoiding the parent upon reunion for a few seconds, and then initiating interaction or contact, a number of infants gave the parent a bright, full greeting (e.g., an approach with bids for contact), then turned away, dazed, and showed strong avoidance. Others showed high distress upon separation, calling and crying for the parent, then turned strongly away or even backed away immediately upon reunion, their faces suddenly expressionless. Others showed the distraught, angry behavior of the insecure-ambivalent infant immediately upon reunion, then unpredictably turned their backs upon the parent and crept strongly away. Thereafter, they exhibited the behavior patterns typical of infants showing strong avoidance.

One of us (blind) was able to identify an abused infant as disorganized/disoriented rather than secure upon seeing her first reunion episode. The infant went at once to her mother at the door, arms up for contact in a full, strong, "secure response"; she was immediately identified as disorganized, however, when she turned away from the door with a confused, puzzled expression, advanced a few steps into the room, and stood with a blank look staring straight ahead. A few moments later, she made oblique approaches to the mother, readily identifiable as the type of approaches which physically battered infants make to adult caregivers (George & Main, 1979). On the basis of her strong, immediate proximity-seeking behavior, this infant had been classified as secure by other investigators.

Another pattern suggestive of temporal disorganization was sudden, undirected out-of-context crying *following* an apparently complete settling by the parent. Many infants cry for a brief period after reunion. Some insecure-ambivalent infants simply refuse to become settled by the return of the parent or through parental efforts toward comfort. Some secure infants continue crying for a period following reunion, but once having had sufficient contact with the parent, settle. The sign that settling is complete is usually that the infant is satisfied to return to a genuine interest in exploration and in play. After this, it is of course expected that the infant will not again become distressed unless there is a threatening environmental change (e.g., mother's second leave-taking, or the stranger's re-entrance).

Some infants who had initially been described as unclassifiable gave sudden, undirected, out-of-context cries following a lengthy period of apparently contented play. These cries differed from those of insecure-ambivalent infants, who neither really settle following the parent's return, nor return to contented play. Because these sudden cries occurred *following* settling and in the midst of contented play, they constituted a disordering of expected temporal sequences. These cries had no apparent rationale within the immediate environment.

Simultaneous display of contradictory behavior patterns. In our review of the literature concerning difficult-to-classify infants, we have already described several instances of the simultaneous display of contradictory patterns. Abused infants were described as creeping or walking toward the parent sideways, or with head averted, or backing toward the parent rather than approaching the parent face-to-face. An infant in our Berkeley sample approached mother moving backward on her stomach with face averted. Other infants in our sample reached strongly for the parent immediately upon reunion but *with head down.*

The impression in each case was that approach movements were continually being inhibited and held back through simultaneous activation of avoidant tendencies (see George & Main, 1979). In most cases, however, proximity-seeking sufficiently "overrode" avoidance to permit the increase in physical proximity. Thus, contradictory patterns were activated but were not mutually inhibitory. One infant both reached for and received objects from the parent with back and arms tense and stiff, stretching forward across a seemingly deliberate distance. One infant approached hesitantly, then backed or moved very quickly away from the parent.

An even more striking example of the simultaneous display of contradictory patterns was *avoidance while in contact with the parent.* This appeared in reunion episodes, often after the infant appeared to be settled from previous distress. Infants who were marked unclassifiable sometimes sat upon the parent's lap – perhaps even comfortably molded to the parent's body – while looking away, either sullen or dazed. One infant seemed extremely comfortable seated on his mother's lap, his body conforming to hers, his arms and hands relaxed. His expression was, however, peculiarly avoidant; he refused her gaze and her vocalizations, and then lightly and incompletely swiped with his hand toward her throat. Another baby sat on the floor for several minutes with her hand upon mother's lap, leaning into her mother but turned slightly away as though to approach the environment; silent and trance-like, she failed to turn completely either to the toys or to her mother. Another 12-month-old had seemed settled by mother and was put on the floor by her side. A few moments later, he had moved slightly away from her to stand in front of her, hands firmly planted on her knees but head and shoulders turned away. He stood this way for several seconds, looking at the floor, face heavy and somber, as though unable to play, unable to interact, and unwilling to let go of mother.

Similar behavior appears not infrequently in classifiable infants, who briefly appear "dazed" upon pick-up, perhaps while recovering from distress. In infants judged to be disorganized/disoriented, however, the behavior appears long after initial pick-up, lasts for a substantial period, and appears contradictory. If the infant is comfortably settled by contact with the parent, why is the infant refusing interaction by silently looking away? And, if the infant would prefer to "avoid" the parent by turning attention to exploration of toys and the environment, why is the infant unable to move out of contact with the parent?

The impression given by avoidance-in-contact is one of the mutual inhibition of systems in conflict; the infant seemingly can neither fully approach the parent nor fully shift attention and move away. While the infant who approaches obliquely at least succeeds in attaining the set goal of increasing proximity to the parent (Bowlby, 1969), the infant exhibiting avoidance while in contact moves neither one way nor the other.

Incomplete, interrupted, or undirected movement and expressions. Incomplete or undirected movements and expressions also appear in "D" infants. Whereas the behavior examples given above referred to disorganization in a mixed or disordered usage of proximity-seeking, contact-maintaining, and avoidance, most examples of incomplete or undirected movements on our tapes involved undirected expressions of fear and/or distress, and hesitant or interrupted movements of approach or of aggression.

Expressions of fear or distress which appear in the presence of the parent, but which involve no physical or communicative orientation to the parent, are one of the clearest and strongest indications of failures of orientation. One infant appeared frightened of the stranger in the second episode of the Strange Situation, as shown by a high, whimpering cry accompanied by downward and backward mouth corners. With no glance toward the parent, she moved away from both the stranger *and* the parent toward the wall, and then leaned forehead against the wall with a fear-face, her eyes opened widely and cast far to the side. A less extreme example is that of an infant who moved away from his mother to the far side of the room during the first reunion episode. Remaining at this distance, this year-old infant suddenly began a full, continuous cry. While crying, he neither looked at the mother, oriented to the mother, nor undertook an approach movement. Rather, he cried while looking straight ahead of him.

Expressions of anger toward the mother appear in infants in each of the three central Ainsworth categories. In each category, the expression of anger takes a characteristic form. Strong, direct expressions of anger are an identifying characteristic of infants identified as insecure-ambivalent. In Ainsworth's original study, infants were classified as insecure-ambivalent because they both sought and angrily resisted contact and/or interaction.

Infants in secure groups can also express anger toward the mother upon reunion, and in our Berkeley sample, infants have occasionally been classified as secure even when an openly frustrated, expressive "swipe" has been taken. For these infants, "hitting at" mother seemed a brief, communicative expression of frustration – often, at being offered a toy when contact was wanted. Finally, while insecure-avoidant infants do not express distress, anger, or frustration openly, sometimes they take a sudden directed aim toward the parent, throwing a toy from a distance, or striking at the parent's foot in passing.

Review of our tapes of "D" infants showed an occasional peculiar usage of resistance. These infants occasionally struck at the parent's face but in incomplete, weak, almost undirected movements. The movements of the infant's hand seemed almost unintentional, or (viewing the video-tape at normal speed) could be interpreted readily as, for example, a merely curious attempt to grasp the parent's glasses or to explore the parent's face or eyes. That these movements were intentional, directed hits at the parent could often only be inferred from careful analyses in slow motion. In one case, there was a sudden, malignant change in the infant's facial expression prior to the slow almost "underwater" movement.

The infant of a "borderline" mother who had recently attempted suicide and who described herself as frequently subject to both homicidal and suicidal fantasies provided an especially strong example of this category. In every respect excepting the unpredictable, interrupted expression of resistance, this infant's Strange Situation behavior fit the "very secure" (B3) Ainsworth sub-category. However, during the second reunion, the infant interrupted his strong approach to the mother with a subtle, avoidant expression of anger. Creeping strongly to the mother, he stopped and briefly turned his head to the side, slapping a toy he had been holding twice on the floor, and then once more slapping his empty hand on the floor in an angry gesture, still with head and gaze averted. He then continued his strong approach and reached to be picked up by mother. The only other signs that this infant was not secure with mother occurred a minute later when, still held by mother, he brought his arm down and across her face in a natural gesture which seemingly unintentionally involved striking her face with a toy. His expression was impassive during this seemingly accidental movement. This movement – consisting of a shift in arm-position for the infant, and a corresponding unintentional strike against mother's face – occurred twice more during this reunion. The infant's face remained impassive or expressed a good mood on both occasions, and the mother also remained impassive. This child was identified as a "D" infant on this basis, without any knowledge of mother's psychiatric or other history.

Approach movements of "D" infants sometimes underwent interruption, hesitation, or consisted of a series of stop–start movements. In a subtle example, one infant leaned toward the mother, but in a slow, heavy manner suggesting that he was resisting and pushing away at the same time. Others approached in an abbreviated, start–stop manner, seemingly unable to make smooth forward movements toward the parent. Two infants who did approach the parent veered away shortly before arriving beside her, and rocked upon all fours nearby her.

Perhaps the most marked example of interruption of approach movements occurred in the infant of a mother who had been both physically and sexually abused in childhood. As her mother approached during the first reunion, this infant had pulled back, winced, and averted her head while kicking angrily on the carpet. Later, as mother again approached and spoke to her, this infant started to lift her head as though to look into mother's face, then quickly bent her head down, kicking stiffly on the floor. After a few more little kicks, she made a sudden hand-to-mouth gesture, froze in movements, and then for the first time reached for her mother, reaching with both arms for mother's leg. However, just before her hands reached mother's leg, and without any sign from mother, she violently pulled her hands back and covered her face with both hands, doubling over as though in pain. As her mother spoke, she twisted far away, then extended one arm toward mother without looking at her, pulled it back extremely quickly, doubled over again, and arched away. (In this single episode, the infant showed several indices of disorganization, namely, interrupted movements of approach, hand-to-mouth gesture, direct indices of apprehension, and simultaneous exhibition of avoidant and resistant movements.)

Stereotypies, anomalous postures, asymmetrical movements, and mistimed movements. These behavior patterns vary from subtle, difficult-to-note facial expressions (asymmetrical movements of the face occurring immediately upon reunion) to obvious and marked stereotypies (rocking, head-banging). These patterns have no obvious orientation with respect to the immediate environment, and may have no obvious stimulus. They are often described as clinical indicators of stress. Many of these patterns are worrisome to observers.

Among these patterns, stereotypies may be the most readily observed. Stereotypies associated with fear or confusion are especially important when they occur at the moment of reunion, or when the infant is held by the mother. An infant of a mother suspected to be abusive repeatedly raised both hands to her ears whenever hugged by the mother.

Asymmetrical facial expressions immediately upon hearing or seeing the parent were observed in three infants from maltreating families. The immediate response to reunion observed in a seriously maltreated 12-month-old infant was as follows (this infant had been removed from home for bruises):

> B hears M's voice and turns and looks to the door. His look is initially blank, brows up some. Looks up at M, averts eyes for a moment, facial expression then divides in two (left vs. right half of face), uplift of left mouth-corner only and wide eyes occur instantaneously as he looks at M, so that for an instant he looks puzzled, disgusted, fearful, or troubled. His face then breaks immediately into an excessively wide smile. (On the next reunion this infant showed a definite fear-smile immediately at entrance).

Mis-timed movements appeared in several infants. One infant very suddenly (and without the usual intention movements) began to creep across the room, moving so quickly that its movements seemed not to be self-monitored in the usual fashion. Three other infants crept across the room with highly asymmetrical movements, one hand slapping against the floor and almost dragging backward as the other hand continued with forward progress.

Freezing, Stilling, Slow Movements, and Depressed Affect. Stilling, freezing, and accompanying "dazed" expressions were perhaps the first "D" markers, which we recognized. Substantial periods of "freezing of movement" (defined by us as cessation of movement in posture requiring resistance to gravity, as ceasing movement for several seconds with arms at shoulder height) and "stilling" (defined by us as cessation of movement in a relatively restful posture, as, falling prone and ceasing motion, or leaning back against the parent, unmoving) identified many "D" infants. Cessation of movement can be seen as a state of disorientation with respect to the immediate environment, or as simple lack of orientation to the immediate environment. The infant usually has an accompanying dazed, somewhat disoriented expression. Stilling, freezing and falling prone upon reunion are illustrated in Figure 2.1.

An infant of a clinically depressed mother exhibited several of these behavior patterns. When mother entered the room in the first reunion episode, she rose, took two steps toward mother, and then fell prone in front of mother in a depressed, huddled posture. At mother's entrance in the second reunion episode, she immediately placed her hands over her mouth, bowed her head, and fell prone again, crying. Held facing mother, legs to either side on mother's lap, she began to move one arm to a position around mother's neck, but then withdrew it and tucked it between her chest and mother's. She then bowed her head and stilled in this posture for 40 *seconds*. Mother assumed a complementary depressed posture, head bowed and unmoving. Parents in several other dyads also stilled or froze in movement in company with the stilled or frozen infant.

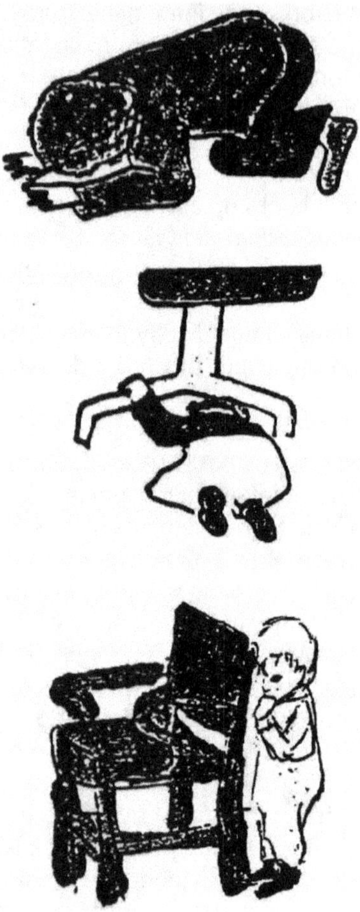

Figure 2.1 Falling prone, freezing, and stilling in 12-month old infants. The infant at the top of the page fell prone in this posture (facing the door) immediately upon mother's entrance to the room. In the middle of the page, an infant stills in a prone posture for several seconds, one hand on a rung of the father's chair. At the bottom of the page, an infant freezes a hand-to-mouth gesture while standing behind the stranger's chair. (Drawings taken from film)

Direct indices of apprehension regarding the parent.[6] Main and Hesse (this volume) have suggested that a state of fear or apprehension regarding the parent (originating in a parent whose behavior is either frightening or frightened) may be involved in the development of the disorganized/disoriented Strange Situation response pattern for many infants. It may play a role in many of the behavior patterns listed in Table 2.1 (as, interrupted approach movements, stilling, and avoiding the parent directly following a greeting). However, in some dyads – particularly those seen in maltreatment or high-risk samples – we have observed more direct indices of apprehension regarding the parent. Once one such movement or expression is seen during the Strange Situation, the observer will often spot many more during the course of the same session. Thus, the infant who is seen to tensely extend the arm toward the parent across an unusual distance is likely also to follow a careful approach with a quick "away" movement, to move apparently casually behind furniture or out of sight of the parent, or to have a highly vigilant or a defensive posture. (At the same time, we have observed seriously maltreated infants who have only one or two such signs, in only one episode of the Strange Situation, as, jerking back from the parent with a fearful expression immediately upon entrance.)

Here, as elsewhere, the observer will want to be cautious in inferring apprehensive movements or expressions. A particularly helpful device adopted by many observers is to imitate the movement or expression of the infant in an effort to understand it. For example, while the words "raising or tensing shoulders when approaching or in contact with the parent" (see Table 2.1) may not have much immediate meaning for the reader, any attempt to play out this movement is likely to suggest the expression of considerable apprehension. Similarly, "mouth corners drawn down and back," when attempted, is likely to suggest apprehension.

Direct Indices of Disorganization or Disorientation. Table 2.1 describes only a few of many direct indices of confusion, disorganization, or disorientation. It is perhaps surprising that "greeting" the stranger rather than the parent directly at the moment of reunion with the parent has been observed in several infants, as has creeping rapidly after the stranger and crying at her departure (first observed in maltreated infants by Gaensbauer & Harmon, 1982). We have also observed two maltreatment group infants pursue the parent, protesting departure, then smile immediately "at" the parent's departing figure or even "at" the closed door.

Directly upon sighting (or even hearing) the approach of the parent, some infants exhibit confusion, in some cases shown in flinging hands and arms in front of face, in some cases shown in a mixed greeting, and in some in a hand-to-mouth gesture (Figure 2.2). One infant hunched her upper body and shoulders at hearing her mother's call, and then broke into extravagant laugh-like screeches with an excited forward movement. Her braying laughter became a cry and distress-face without a new intake of breath as the infant hunched forward. Then suddenly she became silent and blank.

The most marked expression of confusion was a hand-to-mouth gesture (mouth, cheek, or ears) which occurred immediately upon reunion in several of the disorganized infants. One older child had been crying and calling during separation. His immediate response to reunion was disturbing. He bowed his head, stepped backward away from the parent, and put hand to mouth in a gesture resembling indecision, shame, or apprehension. His expression was momentarily fearful. Two of the smaller infants put both hands to mouth and

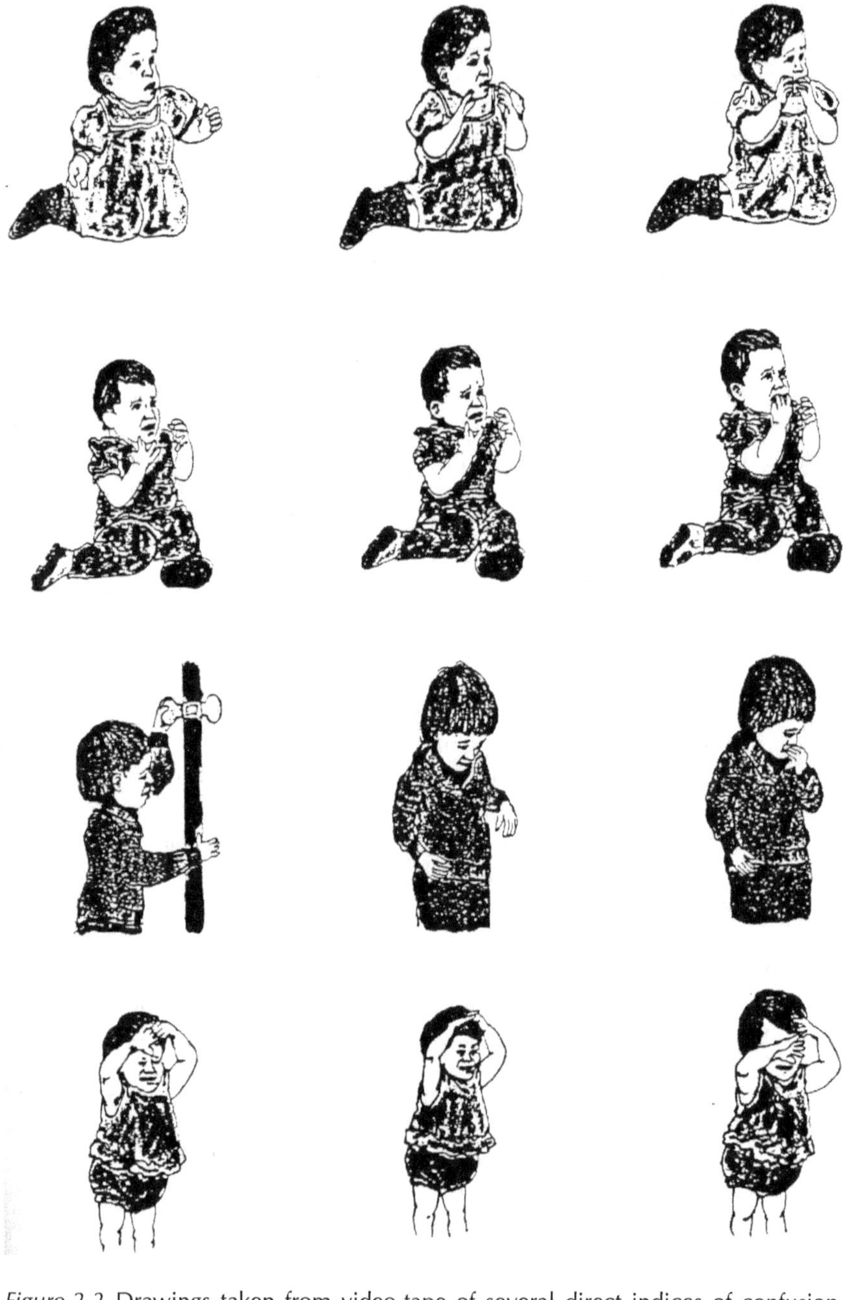

Figure 2.2 Drawings taken from video-tape of several direct indices of confusion, disorganization, and/or apprehension observed at the parent's entrance

cheeks immediately upon hearing the mother's call. The impression in one case was of confusion and in the other confusion mixed with fear.

Several of the direct indices of confusion, disorganization, and/or apprehension observed at the parent's entrance are shown in drawings taken from video-tape in Figure 2.2.

Directions for Determining Whether an Infant Should Be Assigned to Disorganized/Disoriented Attachment Status

This is a list of suggested steps to be taken in determining whether a given 12–18-month-old infant is classifiable, is disorganized/disoriented, or is to be left still unclassified. We specify infancy ages because developmental changes are expected such that relationships which lead to disorganization and disorientation in Strange Situation behavior in infancy later become organized into recognizable patterns. In the case of maltreated children, Crittenden has noted that maltreated children at older ages often develop a compliant, "pseudo-cooperative" response pattern (Crittenden, 1985; Crittenden & DiLalla, 1988). Similarly, follow-up studies using both our own and a South German (Wartner, 1987) sample have shown substantial changes in the reunion behavior of disorganized infants over time, such that the originally disorganized infant often becomes organized into, for example, a controlling-punitive or a controlling-caregiving pattern.

Although we do not know when these patterns of new organization have their onset for disorganized infants, we should be alert to expectable difficulties in studying the Strange Situation procedure for children entering the "transition" between infancy and childhood. We have applied the "D" criteria shown in Table 2.1 successfully with children up to 20 months, but at 20 months, we have experienced some difficulty. Whether this system can be used beyond 20 months of age seems doubtful.

Although some researchers are continuing to classify infant Strange Situation behavior on the basis of narrative records or on-the-spot notations as opposed to video-tape, a quick review of the indices of disorganization and disorientation listed in Table 2.2 will show that these are too subtle for any but video-tape recording. Indeed, the observation of these behaviors takes repeated, slow-motion study of the video-tape. Application of this system (in conjunction with the Ainsworth system) is expected to take the observer between 1 and 2 hours.

Disorganized/disoriented behavior represents a departure both from expectable patterns of infant behavior in general, and from "classifiable" infant attachment status. Although this chapter provides as complete directions for identifying disorganization and disorientation in infant behavior as we are capable of making at the present time, it is more than likely that experience with studies of normal infants and with the traditional Ainsworth system of A,

Table 2.2 Determining whether an infant is to be assigned to disorganized/disoriented attachment status

Step I. Attempt to assign an "Ainsworth" (A, B, C) classification and sub-classification. Infants may fail to fit for many reasons. Two of the more common are (a) reunion behavior qualifies the infant for two major attachment classifications either within the same reunion or across the two reunions, (b) separation behavior is inconsonant with reunion behavior, for example, infant calm and undistressed during separation, but highly distressed and resistant on reunion.

Ainsworth has revised the descriptors for the B4 sub-category to *exclude* "He may show other signs of disturbance, such as inappropriate, stereotyped, repetitive gestures or motions" and ". . . he may avoid (the mother) by drawing back from her or averting his face when held by her." These behavior patterns are more likely indicators of "D" attachment status.

Step 2. Review Table 2.1: Does the infant's Strange Situation behavior fit to any of the specific behavior examples offered – or, does it fit to one of the eight thematic headings while not fitting to the behavior examples ("other")? If the infant could not be given an "A, B, C" classification, but does not appear disorganized or disoriented, it should be considered "U," still unclassified (extremely rare). Infants who show no indices of disorganization or disorientation, but who appear so casually avoidant as to suggest failure to be attached provide one example of still unclassified ("U") infants.

Step 3. Make a written record of all behaviors seeming to qualify as indices of disorganization or disorientation, specifying social, behavioral, and temporal context.

Step 4. If any of these are "pathognomic" indicators (in italics in Table 2.1), the infant is assigned at once to the "D" category.

Step 5. If there are no pathognomic indicators, but one or several other indicators of disorganization and disorientation are present, the worker must decide whether these are sufficient to warrant placement in the "D" category. Take especially into consideration;

a. Whether the infant's behavior seems to have an immediate rationale or explanation within the present context, or whether ("D") its appearance lacks rationale or is inexplicable.
b. Timing. Whether the behavior appears only in the parent's absence (unlikely to be considered disorganized) or in the parent's presence. If the latter, whether it appears before separation (less serious), during reunion (more serious), or during the first few seconds of reunion (very serious).

Step 6. Assign an alternative A, B, C classification including sub-group category. Within any given sample, a "D/C1" infant may eventually be found to differ in experience or development from a "D/A1" infant. For this reason, this information should be preserved.

Step 7. Note whether a tentative sub-classification seems viable. At present, candidates for a D sub-classification include "apprehensive"[5] "depressed affect," and "A–C."

B, C classifications is necessary to this undertaking. The directions given in this section are summarized in Table 2.1.

I. **Attempt to make an "Ainsworth" classification and sub-classification.** Infants who fail to fit coherently to the A, B, or C "Ainsworth" classification (and, for each infant, sub-classification) should be immediately set aside as candidates for "D" or even "U" (still unclassified) attachment status. In the search for D or U attachment status, note any of the following:

a. The infant seems to qualify almost equally well for two major attachment classifications, either by mixing behavior patterns in a given reunion, or by qualifying for one major classification on the basis of behavior observed in the first reunion, but for a second major classification in the second reunion.
b. Be aware of violations of expectancies regarding behavior changes across the Strange Situation as a whole. Specifically, an infant who avoids the parent strongly on both reunions, but cries and calls for the parent in distress while left with the stranger cannot be given an "A" classification. Similarly, an infant who is calm and undisturbed during separation, but becomes distraught and resistant only upon reunion, cannot be given a "C" classification.
c. Ainsworth (personal communication, January, 1985) has revised the descriptors for the B4 sub-category as it is presented in Ainsworth et al. (1978). *Stereotypies, and gazing away while held, are no longer to be considered criteria for the B4 sub-category, but rather are considered more likely indicators of "D" attachment status (indeed, these are now "D" criteria, see Figure 2.1).* Specifically, the lines to be omitted from the current classification directions (Ainsworth et al., 1978, p. 62) are: "He may show other signs of disturbance, such as inappropriate, stereotyped, repetitive gestures or motions," and ". . . he may avoid (the mother) by drawing back from her or averting his face when held by her."

II. **Review Table 2.1, "Indices of Disorganization and/or Disorientation in Strange Situation Behavior": Does the infant's Strange Situation behavior fit to one of the thematic headings described in this table or, more specifically, to any of the behavior examples offered?** For heuristic purposes, the behaviors observed in Table 2.1 have been organized under seven thematic headings: While these seem to us at the moment to be preferable to the many alternatives, different thematic organizations of the many disorganized/disoriented behaviors we have observed are possible.

To make use of this table, the worker should begin by reviewing the thematic headings, then move to the specific behavior examples offered. These examples are useful not only because similar behavior may appear in the worker's sample, but also because they demonstrate the range and type of behavior that to date has been ordered under the thematic heading. By moving back and forth between the video-tape and this table, the worker should succeed in becoming alert to any existing signs of disorganization and disorientation in behavior.

If the infant could not be classified, but does not appear disorganized or disoriented, it should be set aside as simply "unclassifiable." In the

Berkeley sample, two infants who could not be classified were nonetheless not disorganized or disoriented during the Strange Situation. These seemingly non-attached infants are thought to be still unclassifiable.

III. Make a written record of all behaviors seeming to qualify as indices of disorganization and disorientation, specifying social, behavioral, and temporal context. This written record is necessary to determining whether a specific infant is disorganized/disoriented. It is also vital to any future description and development of any coherent categories other than D, and to the development of D sub-categories.

IV. If the infant shows even a single "pathognomic" indicator (indicators given in italics in Table 2.1), the infant is assigned at once to the "D" category.

V. If no pathognomic indicators, but one or several other indicators of disorganization and disorientation are present, the worker must decide whether these are sufficient to warrant placement in the "D" category. Slight indices of disorganization and/or disorientation during the Strange Situation occur in many infants. For example, when left with the stranger during the separation episodes, some otherwise well-organized infants may show slight stereotypies (e.g., hand-to-ears or hair-twisting gestures). As another example, slight dazing (blank expression, gazing off rather than interacting) is not uncommon for a few seconds when an infant is picked up by the parent after a period of hard crying. The worker should, then, expect to meet with occasional "D" behaviors in infants who can be satisfactorily classified. What, then, are the cut-off criteria distinguishing organized infants who are simply slightly disorganized from infants who should definitely be placed within the "D" category?

We suggest that consideration be given to each of the following factors:

a. First, *whether the infant's behavior seems to have an immediate goal, rationale, or explanation within the present context.* A review of Table 2.1 shows that almost all the behaviors listed are inexplicable considering the immediate Strange-Situation context. Thus, nothing in a given situation indicates why an infant would suddenly still or freeze for 30 seconds in the presence of the parent, approach the parent but with head turned backward, fall to the feet of the parent and rock violently back and forth for several seconds, cry loudly while moving away from the parent to the wall, or place hand to mouth at parent's entrance. These are not attachment behaviors; not exploratory behaviors; not behaviors which seem convincingly organized to maintain or increase the physical or communicative distance between infant and parent (avoidance, see Main, 1981); and not expressions of anger (resistance).

b. The *timing of the appearance of "D" behavior* with respect to the Strange Situation. The infant's behavior during the parent's absence is not considered evidence of D status. Behavior during the (third) episode involving infant, parent, and stranger can rarely, but only rarely, qualify an infant for D status. If D behavior is seen in this episode and only in this episode, it must be very frequent, or be pathognomic, to qualify the infant for D attachment status. "D" behavior appearing anywhere in a reunion episode is serious, and "D" behavior appearing in the first moments of reunion is very likely to qualify the infant for D attachment status.

c. *Whether episodes of apparent disorganization* (for example, stereotypies, out-of-context distress, undirected distress) are *immediately succeeded by an approach to the parent,* suggesting some continuing orientation toward the parent and an organized and appropriate use of the parent for mitigating whatever stress the infant may be experiencing.
d. The *extent of difficulty involved in making an A, B, or C classification.* Where this is very difficult, and any of the listed indicators are present, the infant should be considered disorganized.

In making this judgment, we urge workers to err on the side of classifiability (non-D status). A simple 5-point scale can also be used, where 1 indicates easy classification with no signs of disorganization, 2 indicates slight disorganization, 3 indicates some disorganization or disorientation which is not sufficient to warrant consideration of D status. Infants who are determined to be disorganized are assigned a 5 on this "scale," while 4 indicates the presence of substantial disorganization ultimately considered insufficient for assignment to D attachment status. When this or a similar scale is used in combination with the written record of D behaviors, workers can easily re-consider the assignment of infants obtaining a 4 rating to D attachment status.

VI. Assign an alternative A, B, C classification including sub-group category. Each "D" infant should be assigned an alternative "Ainsworth" or "A, B, C" category. In some cases, this will be simple, in others very difficult. Nonetheless, infants who are disorganized may preserve aspects of one of the organized patterns, and this information may be important in understanding correlates of the infant's Strange Situation behavior in succeeding studies. To be explicit, the D/A1 infant may differ in history or in development from the D/C1 infant; since this is not yet known, the information should be preserved.

VII. Among the many indices of disorganization, there are substantial and interesting differences in type. Some infants are classifiable except for freezing or exceptionally slow movement and depressed affect; some are classifiable except for apprehensive movements; and some show characteristics of both the A and C attachment categories.

If we consider, for example, "apprehensive," "depressed in affect," and "A–C" as potential sub-categories of disorganized/disoriented, we will still have difficulty in assigning a particular infant to a sub-category.

Many infants are disorganized without showing behaviors, which fit to any of the above descriptors. There are also often indices of disorganization in a single infant which would permit assignment to several sub-categories, for example, a given infant may appear to be both apprehensive and depressed in affect, or it may show strong characteristics of the both the A and C classifications and be apprehensive.

In some cases, however, it may be that, for example, signs of apprehension, are the only indices, which have led to assignment to the "D" category. In others, the infant may show avoidance and resistance which seem to the investigator to be sufficient to warrant placement in an "A–C" category, without showing apprehension and/or depressed affect. In this case, recording a potential sub-category for the infant may be useful.

This assignment to sub-category should not lead to early reification of these sub-categories. For any potential sub-classification to meet the criteria for a coherent sub-category, we will need evidence for stability or else for predictable and distinct outcome, and evidence for a specific and distinct parent–infant interaction pattern or history. (By distinct, we mean an outcome or history, which distinguishes infants in this D sub-group from other "D" infants). Nonetheless, these tentative distinctions will provide the material necessary to eventual development of meaningful sub-categories, if and where they exist.

"Disorganized/Disoriented"; The Issues of Category Meaning and Category Demarcation

This final section of this chapter addresses the issue of category demarcation. Here, we ask: In what sense is disorganization/disorientation a dimension of behavior which can be seen in the Strange Situation behavior not only of unclassifiable infants but also of infants who can be accurately placed within the three traditional categories? In what sense is it, in addition, a category of Strange Situation response which can be applied to the classification of individuals? Is it also a form of *attachment organization* comparable to the secure, insecure-avoidant, and insecure-ambivalent organizations?

The Ainsworth interactive scales for proximity-seeking and proximity-avoidance offer good examples of the complex but readily comprehensible behavior scaling which can be used in the analysis of infant Strange Situation behavior. Although the behaviors described differ from one another in a literal sense (e.g., looking away from the parent is not the same as ignoring the parent's efforts to communicate), they can all be understood as serving the same function (Main, 1981), and all involve specifically the cut-off of communication with the parent.

It is initially a radical notion that the many, highly diverse indices of disorganization and disorientation listed in Table 2.1 can be placed under one heading. These indices are not similar to one another in any ordinary sense: Rocking on all fours does not look like stilling, and neither of these patterns look like a hand-to-mouth gesture made immediately upon reunion with the parent. If we subscribe to the notion that all behaviors serve a biological function, it is still hard to say what unifying function is served by these patterns. Some of the stereotypies have been taken as stress indicators. However, we are concerned with many types and sequences of behavior other than stereotypies (e.g., disordering of expected temporal sequences), and no theory has been offered to explain why behavior sequences should take one order rather than another, and why one temporal order is to be considered a disordering of expectation. The behaviors do not have even a superficial similarity, and it is only by defining them as disorganized and disoriented that we can hope to recognize them as things of a kind.

It may well be too soon to attempt to offer any theory of a single function served by these diverse indices of disorganization. In point of fact, however, we recognize the similarity of this diverse set of behaviors in terms of what they seem not to represent – these are behaviors which are not organized either to simply increase or to decrease proximity to the attachment figure; not oriented to the inanimate environment in a way likely to increase knowledge of the environment; not organized to decrease proximity to a feared object; not organized to permit social intercourse with persons other than the attachment figure. In other words, these behaviors are recognized in part by an exclusion principle: They are not recognizably behaviors that serve any of the (above) four or five infant set goals described by Bretherton and Ainsworth (1974) as satisfactorily describing infant Strange Situation behavior.

Once we are willing to group them, a simple although not entirely satisfactory rank ordering of individuals can be made. From even the simplest view, an infant who leans forehead against wall and cries in the parent's presence, later interrupts its avoidance with tantrum behavior, and constantly interrupts its approaches to the parent with back-stepping is more disorganized than an infant who stills briefly at the stranger's entrance. This leaves us with the problem of whether there are good criteria for determining if we have on the one hand a somewhat disorganized infant who is still classifiable in the A, B, C system, or instead an infant who should be placed in the "D" category.

The cut-off for the "D" category: "Inexplicable," "unpredictable," "conflicted," or "irrational" behavior. Earlier in this chapter, we suggested that the final and most important question the researcher must address in asking whether a somewhat disorganized infant is a candidate for the category is, whether the behavior of interest can be seen as having an immediate goal, rationale, or explanation within the present context. Whenever, viewing video-tapes of Strange Situation behavior, we thought we could explain the infant's apparent disorganization or disorientation to ourselves (in terms of its easily inferred immediate aims or in terms of the immediate situation), we were satisfied in failing to assign disorganized/disoriented attachment status. Thus, ultimately the infant assigned to D status differs from the infant not assigned to D status in that, during a mild stress situation and in the parent's presence, the infant exhibits (or undergoes) interruptive bouts of inexplicable behavior of a type usually associated with stress or with strong conflict. (Some of the methodological and theoretical difficulties involved in use of this unusual criterion for category placement, that is, use of the observer's judgment that episodes of the infant's behavior are inexplicable or irrational in context, are discussed at length in Main and Hesse, this volume).

As we note below, this explicable/inexplicable criterion for the D/not D distinction successfully differentiated between the reunion behavior of these infants seen during a 5-year follow-up in South Germany (Wartner, 1987). Further analysis suggests that an equally successful distinction can be made between the family drawings of D/not D children in this South German sample, and between the mother–child discourse of D/not D dyads.

In determining that infants were disorganized in infancy, Wartner used not the Strange Situation but rather a rating of "3.5 or higher" assigned on a 9-point scale of disorganized/disoriented behavior exhibited in the parent's presence in a separate, mildly stressful situation (the Clown Session, described by Main & Weston, 1981). The infant was assigned a 3 (or lower) on the scale when it showed disorganized/disoriented behavior, which could be explained by its immediate mood or situation (e.g., lying down because tired, or batting arms up and down because happy and excited). Any infant receiving a rating over 3 ("3.5 or higher") on this scale had therefore exhibited behavior, which could not be explained by immediate mood or context. As we noted above, this explicable/inexplicable criterion for the D/not D distinction successfully distinguished the reunion behavior, drawings, and discourse patterns found in these children 5 years later. Thus, in this cross-national comparison study, the boundary used successfully as a "D-marker" was again whether or not the observed disorganized/disoriented behavior could be readily explained within its present context.[6]

Support for the notion of D as a category. Earlier we discussed why we believe it important to maintain categorical distinctions with regard to infant behavior in the Strange Situation. That is, we believe these distinctions enable us to recognize coherent differences in mental and behavioral organization, which are reflective of critical differences in interactional history. We have now substantial evidence supporting the assertion that disorganized/disoriented can be treated as a behavior category applicable to individuals, that is, that it is meaningful to assert that one infant is disorganized/disoriented in contrast to another who is not disorganized/disoriented. The evidence to date is as follows:

(a) The "inexplicability" of the appearance of disorganized behavior serves as a criterion distinguishing differences in kind from differences in degree of disorganization. Although this is an unusual marker, it is reliable across observers.

(b) We have been able to obtain *inter-judge agreement* with another laboratory using an A, B, C, D classification system, and more specifically to reach high agreement on the D/not D distinction.

(c) We have discovered a *shared background* for "D" infants, that is, the parent's experience of a (still unresolved) major trauma – this background sharply distinguishes these infants from infants who are classifiable in our own and in other samples (Main, 1983, Main et al., 1985; Main & Hesse, this volume; Friedman, 1986; Ainsworth & Eichberg, 1991).

(d) Strange Situation reunion behavior predicts reunion behavior at a later period – that is, as six-year-olds the reunion behavior of disorganized children (seen with the parent with whom they were earlier disorganized) can be distinguished from the reunion behavior of A, B, and C infants (Main & Cassidy, 1988).

(e) The external correlates of the pattern are interpretable in light of our knowledge of the parent's background and our understanding of the pattern itself – that is, the family drawings of these children as six-year-olds can be distinguished from the family drawings of other children, in ways which suggest disorganization, trauma, and efforts to deal with trauma, again in both the United States (Kaplan & Main, 1986) and in South Germany (Wartner et al., 1994); and, the parent–child discourse of these dyads is dysfluent and disorganized both in the United States (Strage & Main, 1985) and in South Germany (Wartner et al., 1994).

(f) All of the sixth-year follow-up studies involve categorical assessments (for example, children's drawings, as well as children's reunion responses are categorized as A, B, C, or D). Thus, it is not merely the case that the drawings, or the child–parent discourse of D children are judged relatively more disorganized or suggestive of trauma than the drawings or discourse of children who were A, B, or C as infants but that the drawing (parent–child discourse) of the D child can again be accurately distinguished from the drawings (discourse) of other children.

"D" seems to be, then, a meaningful category. We should be very cautious, however, in assuming that just because we can obtain inter-judge agreement for D, and just because it has some predictive value as a category, it has the *same* meaning as the A, B, and C Strange Situation attachment classifications described by Ainsworth. The latter have always been seen by attachment researchers as differing attachment organizations, that is, as representing differing and coherent organizations of relationship (Ainsworth et al., 1978; Sroufe & Waters, 1977). Main (Main et al., 1985; Main, this volume) has suggested that these three major categories – first observed in the Ainsworth Strange Situation – stand for three differing systems of *relationship representation* which can be observed equally well in children's drawings, in child–parent discourse, and in transcripts of adults talking about their own attachment histories and current evaluations of their histories. It is not clear that "D" has the same organized, representational status. It may have. An alternative hypothesis is that while being disorganized/disoriented sets any relationship or individual apart, it is not a category of mental representation but rather still denotes the disorganization of some underlying representational category.

Both empirical work and much hard thinking will be necessary in order to select between hypotheses.

Acknowledgments

Mary Ainsworth generously provided helpful commentary and continuing support while we were engaged in developing this expansion of her original system for classifying infant attachment organization. Jude Cassidy, Dante Cichetti, Pat Crittenden, Carol George, Erik Hesse, and Ulrike Wartner also assisted us as we prepared the several editions of this manuscript. Tom Rigney undertook the drawings from video-tape used in Figure 2.2.

We are grateful to the following researchers for permitting us to view their Strange Situation video-tapes: Leila Beckwith, UCLA School of Medicine; Wanda Bronson, Institute of Human Development, Berkeley; Carol George, Developmental Studies Center, San Ramon, California; Vicki Carlson, Washington University; Dante Cichetti, University of Rochester; Clare Friedman, University of California, Berkeley; Mary J. O'Connor, Marian Sigmund, and Nancy Brill, University of California at Los Angeles; Susan Spieker and Kathryn Barnard, Child Development and Mental Retardation Center, University of Washington, Seattle.

We are grateful to the Harris Foundation of Chicago for their support, which made the preparation of which made it possible to prepare the paper upon which this chapter is based. In its earlier phases, the Berkeley Social Development Project was supported by the William T. Grant Foundation, the Alvin Nye Main Foundation, and by Bio-Medical Support Grants 1-444036-32024 and 1-444036-32025.

Notes

1 Krentz (1982) used an "unclassified" rather than a "disorganized/disoriented" title to describe infants who could not be classified using the A, B, C attachment classification system.

2 The Strange Situation behavior of infants in the insecure-ambivalent group seems less well organized to most observers than that of either secure or insecure-avoidant infants. However, within the Berkeley sample, a high proportion of infants for whom the alternative classification was "C" were in fact unclassifiable (disorganized).

3 Originally, we ordered our behavior examples under five thematic headings (Main & Solomon, 1986). More recently, using the same examples, we have developed eight thematic headings. This longer list of headings seems clearer for heuristic purposes (see Table 2.1).

4 This work is still in progress. At present, we have established high inter-judge agreement across a sample of 30 cases, in which at least one judge had determined 17 cases to fall within the "D" category. This first sample was deliberately selected to include infants for whom the "D" classification was given with low or marginal confidence.

5 Signs of apprehension and signs of depression may initially seem less disorganized or disoriented than many of the other behavior patterns listed in Table 2.1.

We would argue, however, that fear of the attachment figure in an attached *infant* necessarily results in disorganization in behavior, because the attached infant will approach the feared attachment figure in a disorganized manner, e.g., approaching with head turned away, or approaching the parent by backing toward her (see George & Main, 1979). (Older children may develop more organized patterns for dealing with an abusive or maltreating parent, as see Crittenden, 1985; and even within non-maltreating, middle-class samples disorganization eventually develops into organization).

6 The scale used in the study of disorganized/disoriented behaviors during the Clown Session in the Regensburg sample may be obtained by writing to the Department of Psychology, University of California, Berkeley, California, 94720.

3 The Adult Attachment Interview

Carol George, Nancy Kaplan, and Mary Main

Guidelines to the Researcher: Ethical Considerations

The Adult Attachment Interview should not be used with clinical or patient populations, or with populations who are at risk (for example, maltreating parents) except and unless it is used by the subject's own doctor, clinician, social worker or counselor. In other words, this interview should not be used as an "intake" interview where the subject tells his life story to one person and then moves to another for counseling. Where this interview is used with vulnerable populations, the interviewer and the helping professional should be identical.

In all cases, some time should be devoted to de-briefing following the interview. The researcher will want to reassure the subject about various issues, including the fact that the confidentiality of the interview will be respected; ask how she felt about the interview; whether she now has anything to add; and whether she now has her own questions. Finally, the interviewer should let the subject know that the interviewer will be available in the future, should any questions relating to the interview arise.

Attachment Interview for Adults

The Adult Attachment Interview is a structured interview, which includes a number of probes. The interview has several unique features. First, it is structured entirely around issues in attachment. Second, it includes features of both the highly structured "questionnaire" interview format and features of the clinical interview. The interview questions are asked in a set order, and specific probes are used when questions are not answered. At the same time, the interviewer follows the subject's phrasing in order to understand what is meant, and repeatedly gives the subject time to answer thoughtfully and to expand upon the topic over the period of the interview itself. Third, it deliberately repeatedly asks for memories and evaluations of experience in two contrasting forms: overall evaluations of experience, and specific biographical episodes. Fourth, the interview is transcribed verbatim, and its analysis depends upon extended study of the transcript as a whole. Much of the analysis

DOI: 10.4324/9781003569978-3

of the interview is conducted through a search for overall coherency in the representation of attachment-related issues (e.g., do memories support, fail to support, or actively contradict more general evaluations of feeling and experience?) and through an analysis of exact linguistic form.

Conduct of the Interviews

To date, approximately 120 interviews have been transcribed and analyzed at Berkeley. The length of the interview (usually, just under to over an hour) depends upon the complexity and number of issues to be discussed, and upon length needed to ensure the subject's comfort insofar as possible.

Practice as "Subject" and With Peers

Learning this interview begins with an initial session as a subject: Before the first practice session in which the interviewer works with a "subject," the prospective interviewer should ask a friend or colleague to interview her. The initial session as a subject reveals the sense of struggle in accessing memories, in selecting words, and in dealing with accompanying feelings, which no amount of observation of this process in the role of interviewer can provide.

The prospective interviewer should next practice with several friends and peers. Some may wish to respond naturally, while some may play the part of particularly difficult, resistant subjects.

Not only should these practice-subjects provide critiques regarding their experiences of the interview, but the interviewer should also listen to the audio-tapes carefully. Obviously, she should be alert to any questions dropped or mis-ordered, opportunities for probes which were missed, or subject responses, which were cut short untowardly.

Memorization

This is an intimate interview in which a natural conversational style and a natural sympathy must be maintained throughout. This is not possible unless the interviewer has memorized both questions and probes. Both searching visually for the succeeding question or probe, and changing topics suddenly in order to move on to the next question precludes a natural conversational style.

Thus, while the interviewer needs to move through the interview questions in the proscribed order, changes in topic and question must not be startling. This can be avoided only through complete familiarity with the interview topics, probes, central aims, and order. The most natural yet accurate interview is probably obtained only when the interviewer has fully memorized the interview, has practiced it, and has available a small "prompt" sheet to be certain all questions and probes are fully covered.

Familiarity With the Classification and Rating Systems for the Adult Attachment Interview

The interviewer should be familiar with both the classification systems and the rating systems which will be applied to the interviews once transcribed. The interviewer need not be prepared to rate or classify the interview, and indeed a mind free of evaluation during the interview is ideal. The purpose of familiarity with the classification systems and rating systems is only that of familiarizing the interviewer with the range and content which will be needed and expected for study.

Efforts to Provide a Comfortable and Natural Conversational Setting

Interviews should be conducted in comfortably furnished, private offices: It may be helpful to the subject's comfort if she is already acquainted with the interviewer through previous interviews or other contexts, and, if refreshments are offered. Because these interviews are audio-taped, there is no need for the interviewer to take notes.

The interviews conducted in our laboratory at Berkeley were not video-taped. Our adult subjects had visited our laboratory several times over the preceding years, and were familiar with the interviewers, who had visited them for an afternoon or evening in their homes a week previously. In all previous visits, however, the child or parent–child interaction had been the focus of study. We decided not to video-tape these interviews in the hopes of alleviating potential discomfort or self-consciousness, and to increase the opportunity for maintaining a natural, sympathetic, and conversational atmosphere. Clearly, some laboratories will wish to video-tape the interview. This will be less difficult for subjects who are used to being video-taped, or who are highly familiar with the interviewer or context.

Where it seems natural or useful, the interviewers may occasionally briefly share their own experiences. This is sometimes useful as a prompt or probe, but also sometimes occurs as a spontaneous sharing of experiences or expression of sympathy. These more personal remarks by the interviewers are not a necessity for all interviews. They should occur only rarely, and should invariably be brief. A check to determine whether the differing styles and experiences of the interviewers affected the Berkeley interviews showed no differences in strength of relationship to the critical outcome variable (security of infant–parent attachment).

Common Errors in the Conduct of the Adult Attachment Interview

The Adult Attachment Interview requires a special kind of interviewing skill: It is, as previously stated, neither a fully clinical interview nor a questionnaire. Interviewers accustomed to either extreme of format may be in special need of practice prior to conducting their first interviews.

Difficulties Contingent Upon Use of a Clipped, "Questionnaire" Format

The clipped, questionnaire format appropriate for many interviews is inappropriate for this interview. The interviewer needs to be continually aware that the analysis will depend upon a study of the subject's exact natural phrasing, not upon whether a particular question is answered positively or negatively. "Yes" or "No" answers to questions are almost useless to this analysis.

Subjects must not be interrupted as they attempt to formulate their thoughts; they must be given time to reflect; the interviewer must have a genuine sympathy and interest and must not hasten to new questions. The subject must be given time to answer thoughtfully, and to gradually expand upon the topic over the period of the interview itself. Secure individuals who are subjected to too formal an interview with too many interruptions or indications that the interviewer is eager to move on to the next question may respond with an understandable reserve, and be mis-classified.

Difficulties Contingent Upon an Overly Informal Style

We have had difficulty in classifying interviews in which the interviewer permitted the subject to wander too far from the topic. Some diversions from the topic by the subject are informative, and should be permitted to the extent that diversion to discussion of other topics will be duly noted and transcribed. Occasionally, however, an interviewer attempts to set a subject at ease by actively joining in the discussion of other topics. This is an error. While the interviewer affirms interest in the subject's responses and gives full time for thought regarding each question, the interview must not become guided by the subject, nor should it become a semi-intimate sharing of experiences by subject and interviewer.

In clinical terms, we would say that the objective of this interview is to "surprise the unconscious" with respect to attachment, through repeated, insistent probing upon the same topic. Few subjects will ever have had occasion to be directly and suddenly addressed with the questions in this interview. The words, hesitations, and phrases found in the subject's immediate response are highly meaningful.

Thus, when the subject is in a position to have to speak immediately in response to, "How would you describe your relationship with your mother in childhood?," mental organization becomes far more accessible to later analysis than when the interviewer joins in conversation regarding other topics, or shares too much of her own experiences. Such moves on the part of the interviewer reduce the potentially powerful linguistic analysis of the interviewer's first, and perhaps somewhat "surprised" response, into the necessarily much weaker analysis of common discourse. Because common conversation follows rules actively developed by both partners, it leads away from potential incoherencies in the representation of attachment.

More specific common pitfalls are as follows:

1. **"Translating" the subject's responses**
   Filling in the last words of sentences; rephrasing responses not as they were but as the interviewer interprets them; attempting to make the subject comfortable through irrelevant and extremely favorable and reassuring re-interpretations of her/his past experiences, when this seems desired by the subject.
2. **Failure to affirm continuing interest as the subject is speaking**
   At times, a respectful silence on the part of the interviewer is warranted, that is, as the subject actively searches for thoughts or for words, or is clearly engaged in personal feeling or reminiscence. However, for most conversations, soft and only semi-verbal acknowledgments of the partner's speech are a necessary component of the listening attitude. They encourage further speech on the part of the subject.

   On the audio-tape, these interjections on the part of the interviewer may be only barely audible as softly underriding without interrupting the speech of the subject. These interjections ("oh," "mmmm," "you went to her?," "ah," "not once?," "I see," "difficult") may not even be conscious on the part of many interviewers; their absence, however, can make the continuation of speech difficult for the subject.
3. **"Cut-off speech acts"**
   This interview is difficult for most subjects. Many of these questions will be addressed for the first time. Therefore, the subject will often need time to pause, stumble, reflect, correct, and think out loud. The interviewer should encourage continuation of the subject's speech through active acknowledgments (above)\and should also listen to her audio-tapes to make certain that they do not contain "cut-off" markers. Some interviewers unconsciously note the end of a subject's first response to an interview question with "cut-off" speech markers, as, "mmHMM!," "uhHUH," "ohKAY."

   These interjections are appropriate only to interviews with questionnaire formats. They indicate to the subject, "Right. We've covered that area, now on to the next." These speech acts indicate the interviewer's desire to terminate further thought and certainly speech on the part of the subject. The natural flow and development of ideas regarding attachment is terminated by these often-unconscious responses on the part of the interviewer. Even worse, the subject understandably feels that what she thinks or feels is not really of interest to the interviewer.
4. **Indeliberate re-organization of the interview format by subject**
   Sometimes, a person begins to answer a question which is to appear later in the interview. The interviewer who is completely familiar with the interview order and questions and who is practiced will be able to allow the subject to speak freely at this point while quickly recalling relevant probes. When this topic is finished, the interviewer can simply add that she will want to be asking more about this topic later. The question should again be raised when

it appears in the proscribed order, with a natural acknowledgment that it has been discussed previously. As an example, the interviewer might rephrase the later question as, "You felt your father was under a great deal of pressure from work when you were young, and that this left too little time for you. Were there any other reasons that he might have behaved as he did?"

Whenever a question has already been partially answered by the subject, the interviewer should actively acknowledge this in first asking the question. A subject who has just explained that she felt rejected throughout her childhood should not be asked, "Did you ever feel rejected as a young child?." Rather, the interviewer begins,

> You've already told me that you felt rejected pretty often when you were little, and our next question is about this feeling. Could you tell me a bit more what you remember about it– the first time you felt that way, and what you did? (etc.).

5. **Failure to probe and "follow-up" on subject responses**
   This is a separate issue from the need for continuing, underriding acknowledgment that the subject "has the floor" and that what she is saying is continuing to be of interest (Item 2, mentioned earlier). Often a subject will make a statement which needs clarifying for the purposes of the interview (for example, responding briefly, "I withdrew" to "What did you do when you felt rejected?"). Clearly, the interviewer needs here to ask what this subject actually did, or how she felt, since "I withdrew" might have any of several meanings.

   In general, the skillful interviewer uses spontaneous probes and follow-up questions more than any other technique in her effort to maintain a natural, semi-conversational style. These probes and follow-up questions indicate that the subject's experiences and feelings are of genuine interest.

Introduction

Our lab has started asking parents about the way they feel the kind of parenting they had in childhood has had an effect on them as parents and as people. So, we'd like to ask you about your early relationship with your family, and what you think about the way it might have affected you. I'll ask you mainly about your childhood, but we'll get on to your later years and what's going on right now. This whole interview will probably take us about an hour.

1. **Could you start by helping me get oriented to your early family situation, and where you lived, and so on? If you could start out with where you were born, whether you moved around much, what your family did at various times for a living?**

   * This question is used both to gain basic data which may be lost elsewhere within the interview, and to establish a relaxed and

conversational atmosphere. At this early point in the interview, the interviewer may feel free to share bits of personal biography or comments, and in the interests of setting the subject at ease, the interviewer may engage in a more normal conversational style (e.g., "I was the eldest with three brothers too," "Was it one of those big farms?," "There was a lot of that kind of thing going on at the time").

- **Did you see much of your grandparents when you were little?** If subject indicates that there were grandparents whom she never met, ask whether this (these) grandparent(s) had died before she was born. If yes, continue as follows: **Your mother's father died before you were born? How old was she at the time, do you know? . . . Did she tell you much about this grandfather?**

* This question functions to inform us whether the subject's parents may have suffered early loss of their own parents. The answer to this question will be important to our understanding of second-generation effects of early loss, but it should appear as a casual and spontaneous query on the part of the interviewer.

- **Were there brothers and sisters living in the house, or anybody besides your parents? Are they living nearby now or is your family pretty scattered?**

* Do not go on to the following question until the subject seems a bit relaxed and oriented.

2. **I'd like you to try to describe your relationship with your parents as a young child . . . if you could start from as far back as you can remember?**

   * Encourage parent to try to remember very early. Many parents say they cannot remember childhood, let alone early childhood, but you should very much shape the questions around starting at least at age five, and gently remind the subject from time to time that if possible, you would like her to think back to this age period.

   * Admittedly, this is leaping right into it, and the subject may stumble. Indicate in some way that this feeling of difficulty is natural, but indicate by some silence that you would like the subject to attempt a general description of early relationships.

3. **Now I'd like to ask you to choose five adjectives that reflect your childhood relationship with your mother. I know this may take a bit of time, so go ahead and think for a minute . . . then I'd like to ask you why you chose them.**

   * Not all subjects will be able to think of five adjectives right away, and, if it seems too difficult, simply permit the subject to choose one or two – adjectives at a time. Be sure to make the word *relationship* clear enough to be heard in this sentence, though without leaning forward and stressing it deliberately. Some subjects do use "relationship" adjectives to describe the parent, but some just describe the

parent herself, e.g., pretty, an efficient manager, as though they had only been asked to "pick adjectives to describe your mother." These individual differences are of interest only if the subject has heard the phrase, "that reflect your childhood relationship" with your mother.

* The following probe follows either the whole set of adjectives, or follows each adjective as it emerges.

- **Okay, now let me go through some more of my questions about your description. You say she was (you used the phrase) _________, Are there any memories or incidents that come to mind to with respect to her (being) ________?**

* Interviewer continues, as naturally as possible, through *each* phrase or adjective chosen by the adult. The interviewer is searching here for specific supportive or illustrative memories and incidents. A specific supportive memory or expansion and illustration are sought for every adjective.

* This adjective choice has proven very helpful both in starting an interview, and in later interview analysis. It helps some parents to continue to focus upon the relationship when otherwise they would not be able to come up with spontaneous comments. However, since the ability to provide either both an overview and specific memories, or only one, or only the other, is important the interviewer must press enough in the effort to obtain these "overview" adjectives that she/he is reasonably certain that they simply cannot be given. Some subjects will protest reasonably that they "just don t like to think that way"; the interviewer should respond jokingly or amiably, ". . . just try! Why don't you start with just one or two adjectives." Not all subjects will be able to provide a full five adjectives.

* In terms of time to answer, this is usually the longest question. Obviously, some adjectives chosen may be almost identical, for example, "loving, caring," and you can cover the succeeding probes for supportive memories on these with one question ("You described your mother as loving and caring. Can you illustrate with some memories?"). "Protective," however, is importantly different from "loving, caring," and the interviewer should seek for separate, illustrative memories. ("You said she was not only loving and caring, but also protective. Any memories on that one?").

4. **Now I'd like you to choose five adjectives that reflect your childhood relationship with your father. I'm going to ask you again why you chose them**

   - **Queries as above.**

5. **To which parent did you feel the closest, and why? Why isn't there this feeling with the other parent?**

   * By the time you are through with the above set of questions, the answer to this one may be obvious, and you may want to remark on that ("I think I know the answer to this next question, but I'd like to ask it briefly anyway . . .").

* While the answer to this question may indeed be obvious for many subjects, some – particularly those who describe both parents as loving – may be able to reflect further on the difference in the relationships through the use of this question.

6. **When you were upset as a child, what would you do?**

    * This is a critical question in the interview, so as much as possible encourage the parent to think up her own interpretations of "upset" to begin with. The variations in interpretation are important, and here again, the first thing the interviewer should do is to pause quietly to indicate that the question is completed, and that an answer is requested.
    * Once the subject has completed her own interpretation of the question, with an answer, begin on the following probes. Be sure to get expansions of every answer. If the subject states, for example, "I withdrew," probe to understand what this subject means by "withdrew."
    - **When you were upset emotionally when you were little, what would you do? Can you illustrate with specific incidents?**
    - **Can you remember what would happen when you were hurt a bit physically? Again, do any specific incidents come to mind?**
    - **Were you ever ill when you were little? Do you remember what would happen?**

    * When the subject pictures going to a parent, see first what details they can give you spontaneously, then ask directly if they were held by the parent, and if so, how.
    * When this series is over, go back and ask remaining questions with reference to the parent whom they have not mentioned.
    * Be sure to get expansions of every answer. If the subject says, "I withdrew", for example, probe until you understand what the subject means by this, that is, what exactly she or he did, or how exactly they felt.

7. **What is the first time you remember being separated from your parents? How did you or they respond? Are there any other separations that stand out in your mind?**

    * Subjects usually give some first memory of going off to school, or camping. However, occasionally subjects will volunteer that they hated separations, or hated having the parent work, asked the parents not to leave – or were relieved at the thought of separation.

8. **Did you ever feel rejected as a young child? Of course, looking back on it now. You may realize it was not really rejection. But what I'm trying to ask about here is whether you remember ever having felt rejected in childhood.**

    - **How old were you when you first felt this way. And what did you do?**
    - Why do you think your parent did those things – do you think he/she realized he was rejecting you?

* Interviewer may need to give an example eventually, but at first give parent a good bit of time to respond to/interpret the question.
* Many subjects tend to avoid this in terms of a positive answer. It may be helpful for the interviewer to give examples from his/her own life with parents. The interviewer should also be prepared to finally cite examples from earlier in the interview when the subject conceivably would have felt rejected.

9. **Were your parents ever threatening with you in any way? – maybe for discipline, or maybe just jokingly?**

   - **Some parents have told us for example that their parents would threaten to leave them or send them away from home. A few of our parents have memories of some kind of abuse.**
   - **Did anything like this ever happen to you? Or in your family?**
   - **How old were you at the time? Did it happen frequently?**
   - **Do you feel this experience affects you now as an adult? Does it influence your approach to your own child?**

   * Many subjects simply answer "no" to this question. Some, however, have reported abuse, or sexual abuse, often suffering much distress in the memory. It is obviously important when the subject is willing to share memories of this kind for the interviewer to maintain a respectful silence, or to offer active sympathy, or to do whatever may be required to recognize and insofar as possible to help to alleviate the distress arising with such memories.

10. **How do you think these experiences with your parents have affected your adult personality? Are there any aspects to your early experiences that you feel were a setback in your development?**

    * Again, in some cases, the subject will already have answered this question. Indicate, as usual, that you would just like some verbal response again anyway, "for the record."

11. **Why do you think your parents behaved as they did, during your childhood?**

    * This question is relevant even if the subject feels childhood experiences were entirely positive. For subjects reporting negative experiences, this question is particularly important. The interviewer may eventually need to prompt the subject regarding some of her stated experiences.

12. **Were there any other adults with whom you were close, like parents, as a child? Or any other adults who were especially important to you, even though not parental?**

    * Be sure to find out ages, whether this person lived with the child, or had any caregiving responsibilities, and the significance and nature of the relationship.

13. **Did you experience the loss of a parent or other close loved one (sibling, or close family member) while you were a young child?**

- **Could you tell me about the circumstances, and how old you were at the time?**
- **How did you respond at the time? Was this death sudden or was it expected?**
- **Can you recall your feelings at that time?**
- Have your feelings regarding this death changed much over time?
- *If not volunteered earlier,* **were you allowed to attend the funeral, and what was this like for you?**
- *If loss of parent or sibling,* **What would you say was the effect on (other parent or) household, and how did this change over the years?**
- **Would you say this loss has had an effect on your adult personality?**
- **How does it affect your approach to your own child?**

13a. **Did you lose any other important persons during your childhood? (Same queries).**

13b. **Have you lost other close persons, in adult years? (Same queries).**

* Be sure that the response to these questions covers loss of any siblings, whether older or younger, loss of grandparents, and loss of any person who seemed a "substitute attachment figure" to the adult or who lived with the family for a time. Some individuals will have been deeply affected by losses which occurred in the adult years. Give them time to discuss this, and make sure to cover the same issues.

14. **Have there been many changes in your relationship with your parents (or remaining parent) since childhood? I mean from childhood through until the present.**

* Here we are trying to find out, *indirectly,* (1) whether there has been a period of rebellion from the parents, and (2) also, indirectly, whether the subject may have re-thought early unfortunate relationships and "forgiven" the parents.
* If the subject does bring up a period of acting up, but it is unclear whether this was real rebellion, probe sufficiently to find out. "Acting up" can be done to gain attention, or to hurt the parents, without constituting a period of real rebellion in the interests of establishing an independence.
* *Do not ask anything about forgiveness directly – this will need to come up spontaneously.*

15. **What is your relationship with your parents like for you now as an adult?**

* This question moves from reflections on the past to the present – the last couple of years, and even this week. Try to find out, indirectly

if possible, how much contact the subject has with her parents at present, what the relationship is like currently, sources of satisfaction and dissatisfaction.

16. **How do you respond now, in terms of feelings, when you separate from your child?**

    * Leave this question exactly as it is, without elaboration, and be sure to give the subject enough time to respond. Subject may respond in terms of leaving child at school, leaving child for vacations, etc., and this is encouraged. What we want here are the *subject's* feelings about the separation. This question has been very helpful in terms of analyses, for two reasons. In some cases, it highlights a kind of role-reversal between parents and child, that is, subject may respond as though it were the child who was leaving the parent alone, as though the parent was the child. In other cases, the subject may suddenly speak of a fear of loss of the child, or a fear of death in general. When you are certain you have given enough time (or repeated or clarified the question enough) for the subject's response, then add:
    • Do you ever feel worried about your child?

17. **If you had three wishes for your child 20 years from now, what would they be? I'm thinking partly of the kind of future you would like to see for your child. I'll give you a minute to think about this one.**

    * This question has proven especially interesting with interviews with adolescents, who often bring up issues regarding the environment, nuclear war, etc. Adults also bring up similar issues (fears of disasters, effect on child or family), and it is of interest to let the subject speak or converse long enough here to see the subject's view of such issues in general. In addition, there is considerable variability in whether the response has psychological elements, for example, "I hope she grows up to feel she can just be herself, and that she likes herself."

18. **Is there any particular thing, which you feel you learned above all from your own childhood experiences? What would you hope your child might have learned from his/her experiences of being parented?**

    * Give the subject plenty of time to respond to these questions. These questions are intended to help the subject use and integrate whatever she has said or remembered within this interview, for her own benefit and the benefit of the relationship with their child.

4 An Adult Attachment Classification System

Mary Main and Ruth Goldwyn

Introduction to the System

This is a system for classifying adults in terms of attachment, based upon an overall conceptualization of attachment in terms of representation. The system is designed for use with transcripts of an Adult Attachment Interview. The reconceptualization of attachment in terms of representation permits the assessment and classification of adult attachment on the basis of language, that is, an exact (verbatim) transcript of the speech used by the adult in the discussion of attachment. While the interview focuses upon the adult's attachment history, it asked repeatedly for evaluations and interpretations. Classification is based not upon individual history, which cannot be known, but rather upon the adult's current state of mental organization with respect to attachment. Thus, it is based upon the adult's overall apparent integrity of thought regarding attachment as seen through a study of speech throughout the interview.

History of the Development of the Adult Attachment Classification System

The Adult Attachment Classification System was developed by studying transcripts of Adult Attachment Interviews for a sample of 102 middle-class adults residing in the Bay Area in California. Each individual in the sample had been seen in the Ainsworth Strange Situation with her/his infant 5 years previously, and infants had been classified following the classification system for infant attachment developed by Mary Ainsworth, though modified to include a separate, insecure-disorganized/disoriented category (Main & Solomon, 1986). Initially, 36 transcripts were studied and commonalities were sought between adults whose infants had been judged to fall within a particular infant attachment classification. Thus, for example, commonalities were sought among all adults whose infants had been classified as extremely avoidant within the Ainsworth Strange Situation, and distinctions were sought between this group of adults and those whose infants had been judged very secure, or insecure-ambivalent within the Strange Situation.

DOI: 10.4324/9781003569978-4

A first classification system was developed from these 36 transcripts. The system was based upon the adult's present state of mind with respect to attachment. In general, among these initial 36 cases, adults whose infants had been judged secure seemed presently autonomous with respect to attachment; adults whose infants had been judged insecure-avoidant seemed detached; and adults whose infants had been judged insecure-ambivalent seemed enmeshed in early relationships. Finally, some adults who were assigned to one of these three categories seemed at the same time unresolved with respect to the mourning of an attachment figure. These adults were most often the parents of infants who had been considered insecure-disorganized/disoriented in terms of Strange Situation behavior.

Setting these cases aside as a development sample, a single judge who had no knowledge of infant classification status (Ruth Goldwyn) worked with the remainder of the adult sample (66 cases). Each adult was classified as autonomous, detached, or enmeshed with respect to attachment. For 48 (73%) of these 66 cases, the adult was classified in the adult attachment category (autonomous, detached, or enmeshed) corresponding to the classification (secure, avoidant, or ambivalent) in which the infant had been placed 5 years previously. There were no significant differences in adult-to-infant classification correspondence (hit-rate) when mothers and fathers were considered as separate samples. Half of the adults had been interviewed by the judge, while half had been interviewed by another assistant. The judge had no information regarding the subject beyond the transcript for subjects interviewed by the second assistant. The adult-classification/infant-classification hit-rate was equally as high when the judge had not served as interviewer. The transcript alone was sufficient to determine the infant classification.

The present, revised classification system is based upon study of the full (102 case) sample. Its development is again based upon a search for commonalities and differences among adults whose infants had developed differing organizations of attachment. The system includes sub-groups. Some of these correspond recognizably to the infant attachment sub-groups distinguished by Ainsworth in her study of infant Strange Situation behavior. For example, infants who had been identified as *secure/somewhat avoidant/substituting interaction for proximity-seeking* in the Ainsworth system (B1) had parents identified as *autonomous/some setting aside of attachment* within the adult system. At the same time, there are more adult classifications than infant classifications.

Procedures for Classification

Adults are given a single classification for the judge's best estimate of current, overall state of mind with respect to attachment. Classification is based upon current state of mind rather than history not only because the facts of history cannot be determined but also because despite diverse experiences of attachment (e.g., a rejecting father and an accepting mother), individuals do seem to come by adulthood to an overall working conceptualization of attachment. At the same time, conceptualization is related to experience, and the adult's picture of her/his history is relevant to the judge's eventual classification.

In making these classifications, the judge ideally begins by reading through the transcript a first time with a view to gaining an overall impression of attachment history, critical attachment events, and the adult's presentation. In this first reading, critical passages are marked, events and evaluations are tied together, and passages or sentences which are particularly striking in terms of language (e.g., incoherent, contradictory, etc.) are noted. The judge next reads the transcript with a view to assigning ratings for the subject's probable experience of the attachment figure on each of the five scales for experience: loving, rejecting, neglecting, pushing to achieve, and role-reversing. For these five scales, separate ratings are given to the subject's experience with mother and with father during childhood (or to other primary attachment figures, if necessary). Difficulties in determining these ratings directly upon the basis of the subject's presentation, "conscious" or "deliberate," are meaningful. A final reading is done to assign the five scales assessing current state of mind with respect to attachment: coherency, idealization, anger, insistence upon inability to recall childhood, and lack of resolution of mourning. (Note: A single overall rating is given for coherency and for insistence upon inability to recall childhood, while idealization and anger are rated with respect to each parent, and lack of resolution of mourning refers to a particular lost attachment figure).

Following the assignment of scores for each of these latter scales, the judge is ready to review the classification system and assign the single overall classification. It is necessary to read not only the sub-group descriptors but also the overall group descriptors before making an assignment, since there may well be cases for which sub-group assignment is difficult. Following an assignment to major adult attachment category, the judge returns to the score assigned for lack of resolution of mourning. If this is high, the case should be assigned both the major category and the further status, *disorganized/disoriented through, loss of an attachment figure.*

Category F

Autonomous with respect to attachment:

Freely Valuing, and Yet Objective

These individuals value attachment relationships and regard attachment-related experiences as influential, but they are relatively independent and objective regarding any particular experience or relationship.

In terms of their reports of *personal history,* individuals falling in this category will either:

- Present a believable picture of one or both parents serving as a secure base or haven of safety in childhood (a picture which is not contradicted within the interview, and which tends to be illustrated through one or more convincing memories of parental giving of comfort or support).

- Or, if parents did not provide a secure base during childhood, they will indicate that they have actively engaged in either a period of rebellion and escape from parents; or, that they are forgiving toward the parents (cognizant of undeserved wrong-doing, and forgiving regarding it); or, that they are strikingly coherent or thoughtful regarding relationships, experiences, and their influences.

In terms of *present state of mind*, these persons often show:

- The ability to take a balanced view of relationships, shown through an ability to be critical of their own part in difficulties in attachment relationships; or the ability to set the parents in relevant contexts while criticizing them; or the sense of proportion and balance implicit in humor.
- A philosophy which includes acceptance of the need to depend on others, acceptance of the import of attachment relations, acceptance of missing and needing others or being missed and needed by others.
- Relative ease with the topic of the attachment interview. Although some individuals in this group protest initially that they cannot remember childhood or cannot describe relationships, these protests are belied by clear memories and/or by thoughtful evaluations. In contrast to adults classified as detached, they do not seem to find the topic foreign; in contrast to enmeshed/ambivalent individuals, the topic seems an open rather than a closed one, that is, these individuals are open to potential alterations in their present point of view.
- Relative ease with imperfection, in the self and in the parents. Acceptance of the imperfection of the parents marks a number of these individuals, and phrases such as "– but I forgave him," "– but I feel at peace with them now" are clear markers of individuals falling in this category. Not all individuals in this category are markedly forgiving, but all are implicitly able to perceive both their own and the parent's imperfections.
- Moderate to high coherency throughout the interview
- Relatively little idealization of the parents. There is little split between the representation of the parents given in general statements or descriptions and what the reader infers of the parents from the interview as a whole and from specific episodes or memories.
- Lack of unconscious identification with the parents. Comparison of linguistic features of the transcripts of adults falling in the autonomous versus the detached and enmeshed classifications shows a strikingly active personal presence in the adults falling in the autonomous category. Asked how she responded to a "rejecting" incident in childhood, an adult judged autonomous might say, "I felt she was being really mean. It really hurt whenever she did that to me"; while an adult judged

detached might say, "You didn't mind it. The mother has to do what is best for the child." Lack of continuing, unconscious identification with the parents – or, correspondingly, the apparent development of a strong personal identity – is a particularly strong marker of the autonomous category.

Within this larger group, several sub-groups may be distinguished.

F1. Autonomous: Some Setting Aside of Attachment

These are individuals with harsh childhoods. These adults share with those falling in the detached category both a setting aside of some concerns with attachment and (occasionally) some idealization of the parents. Some state repeatedly that they have little memory for childhood. They are readily placed in the autonomous category, however, because this setting aside of aspects of former attachment relationships is an active more than an indeliberate process.

There are two sub-groups:

a. Some of these adults have had harsh experiences with attachment figures, but have re-evaluated and re-directed their lives in terms of relationships and experiences (often enough, through actively escaping or seeking to escape the early family relationships). These individuals may have regarded parents and family life as lacking or harsh from early childhood, and may have set out early to find alternative friends or parenting figures. To some extent, early attachments have been simply "set aside" (as is the case with detached individuals) – but these individuals differ from those considered detached in that they attribute effects to experience and have deliberately attempted to create new experiences and new relationships.
b. Others in this group have had harsh childhoods only in the sense of poverty and hard work, in which little emphasis was given to intimate relationships; nonetheless, they retain a mild though unexamined sense of ongoing support from parents. In this case, culture or experience has given little time for thought regarding intimate relationships.

F2. Autonomous: Somewhat Detached

Individuals who are held back from qualification for the F3 category by a slight detachment. This may take several forms. The effects of experience are not fully recognized: or, memory for experience is insufficient; or, a slight fear from an unknown source is present. There may be some idealization of the parent. It may be necessary to return to a study of the general category descriptors in order to distinguish this relatively autonomous individual from one who is relatively detached.

F3. Autonomous

This category is the group exemplar. Individuals falling in this group are highly diverse, and except for sharing a strong coherency throughout the interview, they overtly resemble one another less than individuals falling in any of the other sub-categories throughout the system. For this reason, it may initially be difficult to identify these individuals – while they fit the general descriptor for the "autonomous" category, they may have characteristics of several of the sub-categories.

Perhaps the most striking feature of the transcripts of adults judged autonomous is the lack of idealization of the parents. Speech throughout the interview creates an integral image. If the adult describes the parent as supportive, there are memories of support; if the experience of parenting is described as having both positive and negative features, the reader finds no reason to make an evaluation of the subject's parenting which contradicts the evaluation, description, and summary provided consciously by the subject. (While the subject provides clear descriptions of the negative features of the parent, the subject is not derogatory toward the parent and may be implicitly forgiving.)

These adults may volunteer awareness of personal insecurities, in the present or in childhood. They do not necessarily find all present relationships satisfying. With respect to the inner representation of attachment, however, they have developed either a natural or an earned autonomy. They are characterized by ease and/or by thoughtfulness and meet the descriptors for the autonomous group in general.

There are two sub-groups:

a. Individuals with largely supportive families and childhoods. These may seem less developed than individuals in the second sub-category, because present security and autonomy is a natural function of a secure childhood. These individuals may be simple and clear in their statements, and may initially claim poor memory for childhood or little concern for psychological issues. This lack of memory or interest is belied, however, by relative richness of recall and strong coherency in the actual discussion of attachment. The mark of these interviews is simplicity, objectivity, and clarity.
b. Individuals with difficult experiences during childhood who are presently exceptionally thoughtful. These individuals give the impression of being highly developed. They may answer the initial question with great ease– "Oh, I could write a whole novel about that!" – and/or may have particularly clear memories. Childhood was difficult either in terms of difficulties in relationships (e.g., experiences of rejection or of role-reversal), or in experiences (e.g., loss or separation). Experiences are met with exceptional thoughtfulness, forgiveness, or humor.

F4. Autonomous: Somewhat Incoherent or Dependent

These are individuals who either (a) worry about or who describe relationships in a somewhat confused, not completely coherent way, or else who (b) exhibit an unusually highly developed sense of self, but may seem somewhat soft or sentimental. Often there has been some kind of separation, death, or difficulty in a relationship of which the adult is conscious. This includes experiences of physical or sexual abuse.

There is considerable variation in experience in this category, from individuals whose childhood experiences were largely supportive to individuals whose experiences have been extreme in difficulty. Individuals who have developed some autonomy, but who are understandably somewhat incoherent and confused as a function of traumatic experiences have been placed in this category, together with individuals with essentially supportive experiences who seem somewhat soft, sentimental, or still emotionally involved in past relationships.

F5. Autonomous: Somewhat Resentful/Conflicted

Individuals who are conflicted in relation to their attachment figures, but who are strikingly coherent about it. They may be still resentful or still struggling to please, but they are very aware that the relationship is not ideal, and clear-minded and even humorous despite being caught up in it. The relationship described with the parents is similar to an enmeshed/conflicted relationship, and indeed these adults may have experienced similar types of parenting. A humorous overview is often demonstrated in speech, one that contrasts with the unconvincingly analytical view of the adult categorized as enmeshed/conflicted.

Category D

Detached: Dismissing of Attachment

Dismissing, devaluing, or cut-off from attachment relationships, attachment experiences, and attachment phenomena.

Many of these individuals report little in terms of *personal history.* For individuals placed in the D1 and D3 sub-categories, parents and/or childhood tend to be idealized in the sense described in terms of a positive ideation, which is contradicted by actual memories or by an inability to provide supportive evidence. Individuals in the D1, D3 (and often the D4) sub-groups usually describe the parents as normal or as excellent. However, the experience inferred by the reader is either:

- An experience of lack of closeness or support, in some cases accompanied by occasional silent cruelties – a largely silent rejection; or
- An experience of direct rejection, in the sense of repeated active turning away of attachment; or
- An experience of strong apparent closeness endorsed by the adult to an unusual extent ("wonderful, really wonderful parents") but accompanied by some single or repeated event, which has been the occasion of strong, not fully recognized fears of death or loss.

In terms of the *present*, these are individuals who in diverse ways attempt to limit the influence of attachment relationships and experiences in thought, in feeling, or in daily life. For all individuals but especially those falling in sub-category D4, there is an implicit claim to strength, normalcy, and independence. This is implied in the dismissal of the import of attachment relationships or experiences, or through the dismissal of the potential effects of such experiences.

- Some seem to attempt to dismiss considerations of attachment relationships and their influences entirely from thought or consideration,
- Some seem to speak easily of the negative influences of early relationships, but understanding remains on a cognitive level. Acceptance of the potential effects of such experiences upon present feeling and personality is still missing, that is, hurt and distress are not yet convincingly experienced.
- Many seem to approach the topic of attachment relationships and experiences at an abstract level, remote from memories for actual experiences.
- Actual memories, if accessible, may contradict the abstract "objective" presentation, or may be presented as though told through a third party, that is, as though the self had not been present and feelingly reacting.
- Some seem to experience fear of death or loss without actual experiences of loss, and without recognition of the directive strength or source of the fear acting in present life.

There are three major sub-groups:

D1. Detached: Dismissing of Attachment

Memory for childhood and feeling regarding attachment figures is lost, but evidence of rejection by attachment figures comes up indirectly. The adult seems to have dismissed attachment from his/her mind almost entirely. There is strong idealization of the parent, in the sense of a strong contrast between the semantic picture of the parent as an excellent or entirely normal parent (childhood) and the experience of rejection or lack of support, which can be inferred from a close reading of the interview. The adult has not questioned early experiences.

D2. Detached: Devaluing of Attachment

The adult does not insist upon inability to recall childhood, but an implicit devaluing of attachment and the effects of experience runs throughout the interview. The adult may make strikingly personal or apparently perceptive remarks about aspects of childhood, but a coolness to relationships is evident throughout the interview. Exceptional reliance upon personal strength; exceptional materialism; craftiness or even slyness and manipulativeness regarding relationships may be present.

D3. Detached: Restricted in Feeling

Childhood attachment experiences are not dismissed, and evidence of rejection, lack of closeness, or other unfortunate experience comes up directly (although it may be qualified or contradicted). It is not fully accepted, however, that these experiences have affected present feelings, or the development of the self.

Note: These adults may be moderately coherent in the interview, lacking neither focus nor some objectivity. Incompleteness of a feeling, recognition of personal distress, and incomplete acceptance of the failings of self and parent are the chief difficulties. Otherwise, these adults are close to "somewhat detached/autonomous."

There are two sub-groups:

a. Some picture of the parents' capacity for rejection or cruelty is given, but the individual claims in some way not to have been affected by it, or not really to have been rejected as an individual. He/she may have been, for example, pushed to success by the parents to degrees recognized as untoward – but he/she feels that the outcome was nonetheless entirely favorable. The parent may be seen as having been cruel to the siblings and as having negatively affected the siblings – but not the self, and perhaps the self is seen as favored. Or, the parent may be seen as having favored the siblings unfairly – but, there is a denial of the meaning of this favoritism in terms of direct rejecting relationships between the parents and the self.
b. The adult recognizes rejection or other unfavorable attachment experiences and can speak about them in terms of these having had some influence. Reaction to the experience is still not emotional in the present sense, that is, hurt and anger and missing and depending are still relatively absent and the parent seems emotionally detached from these experiences, even while showing good understanding at the cognitive level. (As opposed to the adult judged "conflicted/enmeshed," these adults are focused and often moderately coherent and objective.)

D4. Detached: Cut-Off From Fear of Loss

The adult is cut-off from some determining fear regarding attachment, that is, unable to determine or identify the source. The adult may remember attachment relations and experiences of attachment as being normally or even extraordinarily favorable. The parents may be described as "wonderful." Sentimental, appealing, or cute episodes or family habits may be recalled. The description of family life may be one of exceptional closeness.

The reader's initial impression of this interview may be one of an extraordinarily favorable childhood – but this impression is gradually belied by the enthusiasm of the endorsement. What leads to placement in the detached category, however, is the adult's fearfulness regarding death or loss, a fear whose source is not conscious. The existence of the fear may be most clear in the discussion of questions regarding separation from the child. It may appear as a theme in other parts of the interview, however; For example, this adult may have always feared the parents would die. There is no "rational" basis for this fear that the adult or reader can determine, since, in fact, the adult had not suffered loss.

Category E

Enmeshed, confused, and unobjective:

Pre-occupied with or by Early Attachments

Confused, incoherent, and unobjective regarding relationships and their influences Passive and vague; fearful and caught; or angry, conflicted, and unconvincingly analytical

In terms of *personal history*, these individuals may report:

- A background featuring a weak parent, usually the mother, who failed in protectiveness. This may have been shown in panicking in emergencies, in general weakness and incompetence, or in an inability to stand up to difficulties, perhaps, for example, to an abusive father.
- In extreme cases, the mother may have "fallen apart" herself during childhood emergencies, so that she herself required concern or care or parenting. The implicit or explicit experience in this case was one of role-reversal.
- This mother, who at the least tended to panic in emergencies (or was weak or incompetent), was not notably rejecting. Perhaps in consequence, it seems simply impossible for the subject to describe the incoherently negative features of this parent.
- If, on the other hand, there were overt child–parent difficulties, they most likely took the form of nagging, perhaps guilt-producing, criticism. This criticism regarding the child's state, accomplishments, failures in duty or appearance seemed undertaken more with the aim of persuading the child to please than with the aim of turning the child away toward independence. The parent needed the child to maintain a particular state or behave a particular way.
- There may have been an emphasis upon family relationships, upon the family past or history, or simply upon the importance of the full, extended family.
- The subject may report having "held feelings in" in times of difficulty, rather than having run outside, shifted the focus of attention, etc. The subject may give the impression of being emotionally stifled.

In terms of *present state of mind*, these individuals differ strongly in terms of sub-group, but may exhibit:

- Seeming inability to move beyond a sense of the self as enmeshed in early relationships, while either accepting this state passively, or struggling against it without success.

- In consequence, lack of development of a sense of personal identity, particularly of an identity apart from that of the family or parents.
- An inability to see the role of the self in any relationship system, or to evaluate the role of the self within relationships (unless with self-deprecation).
- Lack of ability to focus fruitfully, objectively, or incisively during the interview, despite often-extensive discussion of feelings and of relationships.
- These subjects sometimes seem caught up in memories of youth and childhood, or even in current interactions with the parents; at the same time, they seem unable to move "beyond" these episodes, memories, and reminiscences to an objective overview at the semantic or at the abstract level.
- Subjects in this group say something negative with respect to the parent, sounding actively resentful, and then quickly oscillate to a more positive viewpoint.
- In the present, the subject may still be struggling to please the parents; or may seem enmeshed in guilt regarding the parents; or may be struggling unconvincingly to prove an independence of identity.

There are three sub-groups:

E1. Enmeshed: Passive

The most striking feature of this interview is the implied passivity of thought processes regarding an ill-defined experience of childhood. The reader has the impression that there was an inchoate negativity in this adult's childhood, which did not take the form of parental rejection (in the sense of the parent turning the child away toward independence). Speech during the interview may wander to irrelevancies, or become confused, vague, or incoherent. It is difficult to determine this individual's experience of childhood, but it is likely that there was enmeshment of relationships, and some emphasis upon the past or upon the extended family.

At the present time, this individual may have a vaguely good, even hallowed memory of his/her childhood, and this is not (cf. D4) accompanied by fears of loss. The individual may be caught up in hallowed memories of parenting and of the past in general.

If, on the other hand, there are some negative descriptors of parenting, they are not used meaningfully to create a coherent picture of parenting and may disappear in contradictions or irrelevancies. If there has been a struggle for independence in this individual, it is limited or has remained inaccessible to awareness.

E2. Enmeshed: Conflicted and Ambivalent

The individual recalls unfortunate early attachment experiences, though these cannot be described as memories of rejection. The subject may recall an incompetent or weak mother, who failed to stand up to an abusive father; or, a mother for whom the subject was excessively important; or a mother who had a child-like response to emergencies and herself required to be parented.

This individual is now hurt and caught up in a still-continuing dependency, or angry and struggling consciously for independence.

While the detached-restricted adult gives the impression of a coherent recognition of their potential cause without a feeling of awareness of the impact of these experiences, individuals give the impression of being aware of affects without being able to coherently identify them. At the same time, there may be an air of authority regarding the effects of past experience, or the individual may be exceptionally talkative and pseudo-analytical. Speech regarding experience and its effects may be highly pseudo-psychological. The individual may impress the reader as particularly egocentric.

E3. Enmeshed: Fearful

This individual has had fearful attachment experiences – for example, experiences of physical or sexual abuse, traumatic loss, psychosis in a parent, or simple cruelty. There is evidence within the interview of an active struggle with these experiences, but the subject is still implicitly fearful, confused, or overwhelmed. The subject is not yet objective, or able to gather these chaotic and fearful episodes of experience into a single abstract yet personally meaningful form.

Experiences of the Parents in Childhood: Loving, Rejecting, Pushing to Achieve, Neglect, and Role-Reversal

These five scales are used to reflect your best estimate of the subject's experience of the parent. This may differ from the subject's estimate, and may be based upon your interpretations of the transcript rather than upon the subject's own direct presentations.

Rate both the subject's mother and the subject's father on each of these scales. All scales are 9-point scales.

Why is there only one, over-arching scale for "loving," but four scales for negative experiences? Because, as Tolstoy states in the opening lines of Anna Karenina, "Happy families are all alike, but each unhappy family is unhappy in its own unique way." The degree to which the subject experienced love, interest, care, support, and acceptance can be expressed on a single scale. But difficulties differ. One unloving parent may have pushed the child to achieve but never have left it neglected; another parent may have needed care by the child so badly that the child felt completely responsible for the parent's care, yet there may have been no push to achievement by the same parent, and little rejection; another parent may have been absent throughout most of the child's life, hence neglecting, but may have been actively accepting when present.

Loving Versus Unloving Parenting in Childhood

This scale assesses the extent to which the subject, in your best judgment, experienced mother or father as loving or unloving in childhood. It is based upon a thorough consideration of the transcript, in which the subject's descriptions, evaluations, and memories are balanced against one another to achieve a final sense of the subject's experience. The central question is whether the subject had a firm sense of emotional support from the parent, a parent who could be essentially trusted in times of trouble, and whether the parent was in addition actively loving.

Where there is little love experienced with a parent, there may have been simply a lack of interaction or any positive experiences; or the parent may have been actively rejecting, neglecting, pushing the child to achieve to a degree that risks mental or physical health, or demanding of parental care herself. The reader of the record may well find this information only through indirect evidence. Many subjects who seem to have experienced little or no love from the parent describe the parent as "loving" in response to the first request for adjectives, or answer "yes of course" to the question "Was your parent supportive?" (Note: A very low rating can be given where a parent gives highly acceptable physical or even educational care without affection.) The parent who is rated as unloving may not actively reject, neglect, or need care, etc., but the parent may still be given a rating of "unloving" if there is simply no evidence for any kind of affection beyond the parent's presence, and support in terms of education and physical care.

The subject whose parent receives a 5 on this scale has an average, and on the whole "good-enough", experience with the parent. While the parent may have been disappointing in terms of being especially affectionate or especially noting of the child as an individual, the parent was not lacking in average care and interest. The parent may have simply been adequate in most ways, or may have had unloving, unaffectionate aspects, which were balanced by behavior or responses in other areas. A rating of 5 indicates that the parent was neither especially loving nor especially unloving toward the subject in childhood. There is a sense of missing out, but not of having had experiences which could potentially be distorting.

The subject whose parent receives a high rating on this scale experienced a parent who was actively loving and accepting, and who had a continuing healthy dedication to this child and his/her development. This does not mean that the parent was perfect. The parent may have been a bit over-protective, may have pushed a bit here or there, or may have had an occasionally explosive temper, or there may have been a period of mismatch and rubbing on one another's nerves. The especially relevant statements and memories here are as follows (always presuming that they are believable, and are not contradicted elsewhere in the record):

- Direct statements such as the following, especially when they are "volunteered" rather than appearing in response to a particular question:

  "I always knew my mother was there for me, no matter what, and I could depend upon it."

  "I acted up a lot, but I always knew I'd get forgiven."

In their thoroughness, directness, length, and clarity these statements would indicate the experience of a loving mother, in a way that "She was dependable" or "She was supportive, of course" does not.

- Memories of physical love, comfort, or affection, such as the following:

being held or hugged for comfort.
cuddling together, napping together.
being regularly taken onto a lap, or having a special time of day when close affection could be expected.

- Memories of having done something bad, or which the child expected to be bad, in the eyes of the parents and being loved or supported instead of scolded.
- Memories of having done something bad or having "acted up" repeatedly in view of the parent, with the expectation of being both scolded and ultimately forgiven.
- Memories of having done something bad in the eyes of teachers or other authorities or adults and being supported by the parents.
- Memories of having experienced childish or childhood fears and being comforted or supported.

1. *Very Lacking in love*
The parent was not at all emotionally supportive of the child, or interested in the child as an individual. The parent was very rejecting, neglecting, pushing to achieve, or demanding of parental care from the child, or showed some combination of these qualities at less extreme levels. The parent may have been actively frightening, or completely withdrawn. Perhaps the child could not go to the parent when hurt, either for fear that the parent would fall apart herself, or for fear that the parent would be angry.
Give this rating also when there is simply no evidence of any real affection or interest, even when high scores cannot be given on any of the "negative" scales. (Note: The parent may nonetheless have fed the child, kept the child in good clothes, and provided education.)
2. *Lacking in love*
The parent may have been mildly supportive, but there was no personal caring or interest or affection that is convincing to the reader. There is a sense of a mild but inadequate supportiveness, or perhaps of bouts of real affection which cannot really compensate for neglect, rejection, or excessive pushing for achievement. All active indications of a loving childhood listed above are absent from the record. (Note: The subject may nonetheless state that parenting was fine or normal.)
5. *Neither unloving nor actively loving*
Support, concern, and interest were probably present, and hence the child probably received "good-enough" parenting. Dedication to the child as an individual, and special memories of love or feelings that the parent "was

always there for me. No matter what" are absent. Perhaps the parent was hard-working, and the subject was one of several children. Or perhaps the parent had negative qualities, which were balanced by affection or an essential trustworthiness, for example, a parent who was frightening at times or absent for long periods but who was essentially trustworthy or who was loving when present.

7. *Loving*

   The parent was loving and accepting of the child during childhood, even though in addition there may have been quarrels or problems. The subject describes this experience directly, and although problems may also be described, the essential love within the relationship is not contradicted within the record. The subject has some memory or makes some statement of the type listed earlier.

9. *Very loving*

   The parent was not only very loving and accepting, but had in addition a healthy dedication to this child and his/her development. The subject has loving memories of the parent and was clearly cherished. This does not mean that the parent or the relationship was perfect. The parents may have pushed, restricted, or acted unwisely here or there, and the subject may readily describe these difficulties and their influence. But there are real incidents to support the notion that the child could count on the parent; that the parent actively cared for and supported the child; and that the parent treasured the child and found pleasure in her.

Rejection: Aversion to/Avoidance of the Child Or the Child's Attachment

This scale assesses the extent to which the parent rejects and/or avoids the child's attachment, or even avoids or rejects the child herself in her entirety. For the most part, what is meant here is a cool rejection, which need never involve abuse in behavior or in language. The essential quality being assessed as rejection is the quality of "turning back or away" (from the Latin *re-jacio*) from the child and the child's affection and attachment. What is expected of the child is probably independence.

At the low end of the scale, the parent may simply have placed a somewhat early or inappropriate stress upon independence, perhaps urging the child not to cling while simultaneously urging the child to acquire skills and achievements too early. At the mid-point of the scale is the parent who is reserved, cool, stern, or inexpressive, but not beyond the limits of what would be expected for some cultures at times, for example, Puritan New England. At the high end of the scale, the parent's behavior is indicative of a real and pervasive turning away of this specific child. The parent seems not to have wanted the child, and to express this through more than mental or physical absence; there is an implication that the parent would either actively like to be rid of her, or that the parent is emotionally abandoning even when present.

The following are signs of rejection of attachment:

- There are no *voluntary* remarks during the interview on expressions of physical affection from the parent, although the subject may answer "Yes. Of course" to "Did the parent hold you?" or even add "I'm sure she must have taken me on her lap." But these remarks are unconvincing in the context of the interview as a whole, or they are contradicted.
- The subject responds that when upset, she kept to herself, or went away.
- The subject *avoids discussing* the *relationship* with or to the parent, although she may state repeatedly that "it was fine."
- The subject begins to recount an incident of being hurt or upset, or an incident intended to demonstrate parental supportiveness, but the incident has an odd ending, or no ending, and does not demonstrate support.
- The subject remembers active rejection by the parent – degrading or abusive treatment, being told to leave, etc. – or else recalls a childhood that was empty of affection.
- The subject remembers rejection of siblings, directly or by implication, without showing *convincingly* that she/he was an exception.
- The subject recalls *serious* threats of abandonment.
- The subject recalls being picked at, criticized, nagged (this is not necessarily strong rejection – the critical parent may be pushing or picking at the child, but not really turning her away).
- The parent was *angry* with subject when subject hurt herself (be sure to distinguish this from "upset" or "panicking"). This is an indication of strong rejection of child/attachment.

1. *Not at all rejecting*
   There is no indication at all of rejection of the subject during childhood. The subject may recall disagreements or "spats," but these do not seem associated with rejection. The parent may have been entirely supportive of the child and extremely loving. Alternately, there may have been some difficulty in the relationship such as strong role-reversal, with the parent actively utilizing rather than turning back the child's dependence.
3. *Slightly rejecting*
   Either a brief period of rejection or a slight sense of rejection (as in an early push to independence or achievement) seems to have been experienced by the subject, but it does not seem to have played an important role within the representation of the relationship.
5. *Moderately rejecting*
   Perhaps the child is seldom given any encouragement, or told that the parent is glad to have her around, or proud of her. The parent may be reserved, removed, or physically cold, or "stern." This parental "remove" does not go beyond culturally accepted limits, however, and might not be uncommon in essentially supportive parents living within some cultural settings. The rejection goes beyond early stressing of independence, push

to achievement, or single brief periods of childhood. The parent's affectional response to the child is consistently somewhat limited.

7. *Rejecting*
This parent is more than reserved, aloof, or removed and business-like. Absence of tie or closeness between subject and parent is an impressive quality of the interview as a record, and rejection of the child has become a pervasive quality of the relationship. Rejection is definite; however, there is no indication that the parent would have preferred to be rid of the child entirely.

9. *Very rejecting*
There seems to have been no emotional tie at all between this child and parent. There is no indication of support, and there may be indications of emotional abandonment. The reader may have the impression that there was an active dislike of this child, or that there were quiet emotional cruelties. The child and the child's affection were turned away entirely. The reader may infer that throughout the child's life, the parent desired/preferred her absence.

Neglect: Physical Absence/Inaccessibility Or Psychological Unresponsiveness

This scale deals with the parent who is inattentive, pre-occupied, otherwise occupied, uninvolved, inaccessible, absent. This may be because the parent must manage a large or busy household; is working a large or time-consuming family business; is often away or was away for a long period of time during childhood; or is at home but depressed or ill or otherwise withdrawn psychologically. At low levels, the child simply misses out on play, interaction, or conversation. At high levels, the child misses out on having a parent.

The strongly neglected child grows up, or attempts to grow up in a psychological void with respect to the neglecting parent. There is a lack of connection with this parent, and in consequence, the child's needs, interests, failures, and achievements go not only unsupported but also unnoticed.

Neglect as defined for the present scale means absence, physical or psychological. A parent, who actively responds to the child, even in a distorted way, is not considered neglecting of the child insofar as there is responsiveness. Neglect is easily distinguished from a push to achievement. It may be useful, however, to consider the ways in which it is to be distinguished from rejection and role-reversal.

Distinguishing Neglect From Rejection

The child who is neglected may or may not be simultaneously rejected. Even in fairly strong cases of psychological or physical inaccessibility, the child may feel more unnoticed than noticed, disliked, avoided, and rejected as an individual. The problem with the parent who is neglecting rather than rejecting is probably felt as being less individually directed. If the parent is absent or ill, the child may be aware that the whole household suffers from the parents' inaccessibility, so that the child and household together have missed out on something, but the child may not have felt mistreated as an individual. "He was almost never home, and when he was home he only had time for my brothers." seems to imply rejection as well as neglect. "He was seldom home, but when he was he was gentle and warm with me." is neglect but definitely not rejection.

Distinguishing Neglect From Role-Reversal

The neglecting parent may or may not be role-reversing. The parent who is neglecting out of being pressed and busy may well not be at all role-reversing. Indeed, as with poor or immigrant families, the parent may have little time for interaction with the child simply because of struggling so hard to be a providing and responsible parent. The depressed or sick parent may also be neglecting without role-reversal (although this may be harder for parent and family to manage). This is most likely if older members of the family make clear that the parent's illness is primarily their responsibility, and the parent herself makes clear her psychological care is not up to the child. Such a parent may be seen seldom (as an ill parent living at home). While the child may help with meals or the household, the child's helpfulness in this case can conceivably be seen as a source of pride, or grown-upness, rather than as an index of role-reversal. It is not seen as role-reversal if it is needed physically, but not needed psychologically, by the parent.

Indices of neglect:

- Although home much of the time, the parent is pre-occupied with work, or the family business, or too large a household.
- Although home and not pre-occupied with other concerns, the parent is somehow unable to care for the child, perhaps because this simply seems "too much" for her, or because the child is expected to care for the parent, or because of depression or illness.
- Parent is absent from the home (perhaps being away at war, or ill, or has divorced the other parent).
- Subject states that parent "just didn't seem to have much time for me." If this is contrasted with a sibling, it is definitely not only neglect but also rejection.
- Parent traveled a great deal, for business or for pleasure.
- There was a major child–parent separation, or repeated separations.

1. *Physically accessible and psychologically accessible in the sense of being positively OR negatively responsive*
   The parent is almost always present and responsive. There is no felt lack of attention, although there may be too much attention, or the wrong kind of

attention. The parent may be pushing the child, or rejecting of the child's initiations, but the parent is definitely responsive.

3. *Mildly inattentive, or absent somewhat more than desirable*
   The parent is mildly inaccessible. This may be because, for example, the parent has to travel in conjunction with business, or works long hours, or because the parent is managing a large and busy household. In consequence, the child misses out on play or interaction or attention, but this is not continual, and the parent is still essentially accessible.
5. *Definitely inattentive, or absent for long but restricted periods*
   The rationale for the parent's inattentiveness may be similar to that presented earlier, but it is on the verge of being a problem The parent may still be uninvolved with the child only because of lack of real and present work investments, or a large household, but lack of an ideal amount of interaction is becoming a lack of sufficiency. The parent may also be psychologically unresponsive to the child because of mild depression, some incompetence as a parent, or role-reversal, and be insufficiently responsive in consequence. This rating would also be given where a parent was absent for some period, but was not at all neglecting once re-united with the family (as a parent returning from war). For this rating, the parent still would not quite be called actively neglecting. This amount of neglect is no more than what might be expected in many cultures or situations, for example, an extremely hard-working immigrant family, or one in which the father has been away at war.
7. *Neglecting*
   The parent is definitely physically or psychologically neglecting. If present in the household, the parent is unresponsive for long periods. If absent from the household, the absence is long, or it is repeated, so that the parent misses some of childhood. Parent and child are beginning to be unknown to one another. However, the parent is not completely psychologically absent, or the long physical absence is followed by real interaction and parenting. This is the rating most likely to be given for a depressed parent; for a parent who completely abandons the child in favor of work; and for a parent repeatedly absent.
9. *Strongly neglecting*
   The parent has almost nothing to do with the child, physically or psychologically, for a long period of time, or for repeated periods. Perhaps the parent was away throughout the subject's childhood, or was repeatedly away for long periods, while being pre-occupied while present. Perhaps the parent was physically present but completely inaccessible and inattentive.

Pushed to Achieve in Childhood

This scale assesses the extent to which the child was pushed to achieve some particular status or position or pushed to exceed other children in childhood. At the low ends of the scale, the parent may be concerned with grades or school performance to an extent that made the child uncomfortable at times, but not beyond reason. Perhaps report-card time was worrisome in terms of disapproval or talking-tos, but the child did not feel a continual push at other times. Or perhaps, again at low ends of the scale, the parent's pushing came from protectiveness which had to do with the feeling that "it's a rough world out there, and a child needs to be prepared with a good record." At the low end, too, if hard work was expected from the child (e.g., in the fields, in a poor family), it was expected because it was vitally needed for family survival, and there are no indications it was connected to punishment or withdrawal of an emotional relationship.

At scale mid-point, the child carries a burden which is not only placed upon her for her own good in facing the world, or for continued survival of the family but also for what she can do to *advance* the status of the parent (the parent's feelings of worth and status). This moves into a realm in which achievement or failure to achieve (or, in an alternative scenario, hard work or failure to participate in hard work) affects the child–parent relationship. The child's daily status vis-à-vis success in the outside world is assessed with a continual watching of performance. Or, if the child's achievement is to be in hard work more suitable for adults, there is implication that what is expected goes beyond what is needed for the family, and is becoming bound up into the relationship. Nonetheless, at scale mid-point, the parent probably feels much better about the child when the child does well, but does not truly withdraw from the child when she fails.

At the high end of the scale, the relationship is maintained or flounders on the basis of the child's achievements. Perhaps the child was to be a famous pianist, with no wish to be one, and was pushed to the stage in the interest of the parent. Perhaps the child was simply urged and forced to be a success in life, in a way that could have risked physical or mental health. This could also be done in terms of forcing the child to work as an adult, with no release, and *beyond* direct necessity for the family. There is no question but that the parent would have withdrawn affection from the child if the child failed. (The child may however, have succeeded, and this may still be the basis of the relationship to the parent now in adult life.)

"Pushed to achieve" must be distinguished from (a) simply discouraging attachment behavior, which is rejection, or (b) asking the child implicitly or explicitly to act as a parent to the parent. As an example, simply being encouraged to keep hurts and disappointments to oneself, or not being able to talk with the parent, has no bearing on this scale, while being expected too early to take physical care of oneself, or to drive a car while other children are riding bicycles, does. Thus, two sorts of parental behavior, which might in each case be called pushing the child to independence, are in the one case rejection, and in the other pushing to achievement. These may or may not exist side by side in the same parent.

Asking a child to manage a household on her own too early is pushing to achievement, but it may well not at all include psychological role-reversal.

The point to role-reversal is that the child is implicitly or explicitly to *psychologically* parent the parent, or at least to worry about the parent's well-being. A child can be asked to take care of a household, or all the little brothers and sisters, thus *replacing* the parent, without being asked to turn directly toward the parent and worry about her. In this position, the child may be experiencing rejection rather than role-reversal.

The following are signs of pushing the child to achievement:

- Report-card time always caused anxiety.
- The subject says the mother or father "always encouraged us to take care of ourselves" in terms of managing the house, feeding selves, and other duties normally taken over by parents.
- The parent encouraged the subject to "get out there and show 'em." This could be in terms of exceeding in school, or in terms of being macho (fighting), or in some other terms.
- Intellectual excellence was stressed from early in childhood.
- The child was asked to do a man's or woman's work early.
- The child was expected to have a career, early; or not only to be excellent but also to stand apart from others.
- Subject stresses push to achievement in family that this was too much for some siblings, or too much in general is implied, and even that it was enough to break health. Subject may or may not have "made it" personally.

1. *Encouraged or not encouraged to achieve, but definitely not pushed to achievement*
   The parents may be proud of the child's achievements, and yet this does not affect the relationship. There is every reason to believe the child would be supported lovingly in failure. The parent may or may not encourage the child to achieve actively, but if the parent does actively encourage achievement, it is in terms of sharing with the child a child's natural wish and the need to do well.
3. *Slightly pushed to achievement*
   The parent is a bit overly concerned about achievement throughout childhood, or for a restricted period, or pushes strongly over some restricted single issue. Grades may be too serious a matter for a while, there may be too much concern at report-card time, or the parent may push the child to work for the family a bit excessively. All this may be shown directly, with reference to the subject, or the subject may simply refer to what was expected of "*us*" and have felt adequate or inadequate. Still, for this rating, the parent did not act beyond reason for any extended period of time.
5. *Moderately pushed to achievement*
   Achievement is beginning to be worked into the fabric of the relationship, but the essential atmosphere of the family and this particular child–parent relationship *may* still be loving. Perhaps the parent's own sense of status rests too much on the child (as in the classic nineteenth-century immigrant

family, a farmer who wanted to be proud that his children started helping in the fields at an earlier age than other children). The parent probably feels better about the child when the child succeeds but does not truly withdraw from the child when the child fails. Nonetheless, the push to achieve is becoming a painful memory, and/or was distinctly excessive.

7. *Pushed to achievement*
   The push to achievement is exceeding the bounds of the norms of almost any culture, and lack of achievement is an occasion for withdrawal of relationship. The child is beginning to feel that his/her importance rests on success (though of course in the subject's report this may not be directly stated). The child may not yet be being punished for lack of achievement and the parent may just "go cold" in response.
   The parent will, however, definitely make the child feel inadequate for lack of achievement. However, for this rating as opposed to higher ones, there is no indication that the child would have been pushed to the breaking point. There was a limit at which concern for the child overrode concern for the child's achievement.
9. *Pushed potentially to breaking point in terms of achievement*
   There are implications that the child was pushed to the point where mental or physical health could have broken. That parents have stressed achievement to this degree is unlikely to be directly stated by the subject. The subject may refer to siblings, who "could not take it" or may refer to this condition very lightly.

Scale for Role-Reversing Experience in Childhood: Parent is a Concern to or Is in Need of Care by the Child

This scale deals with the extent to which the parent's psychological or physical well-being was a concern to or responsibility of the child, that is, with the parent's implicit or explicit need for care by the child. At the low end of the scale is the parent who is either slightly incompetent or slightly over-protective, so that the child has to worry about her worrying. At the scale mid-point, the parent is incompetent or inadequate; or the child feels some implicit responsibility for the parent; or the parent may directly make clear that the child should attend to the parent in some ways, but still the parent is parental in other ways and does not really reverse roles with the child. At the high end of the scale is true role-reversal. The child feels responsible for the parent's welfare, and the parent unquestionably has the role of the child.

Perhaps the assessment can be better understood if we review the reasons that the parent might be a worry to the child. At the low end of the scale, there is simply the "worrying" parent *or* the slightly incompetent parent. *If* we can assume (as we do in giving this a low rating) that the parent can be parental when and where it counts, this faint incompetence or excessive worry about the parent worrying probably has little pervasive effect on the development of the child.

At scale mid-point, either the parent is strikingly incompetent, inadequate, or the child's attention to the parent's needs is beginning to be woven into the relationship, that is, the parent's care for the child is beginning to be implicitly bought at the price of the child's commitment to attending to the needs and concerns of the parent. Nonetheless, the parent is probably still competent when the child is hurt, may be quite competent in general, and can be relied upon in many ways. The implicit demand for care and concern is probably no more than to be expected in cultures in which children are encouraged to care for and be involved with parents throughout their lifetime.

At the high end of the scale, the parent is unlikely to be at the norm in any culture. He or she is likely to be emotionally at the edge of breakdown; the house may be in chaos; and/or the parent may actually be physically or mentally ill. Here, the child must worry not merely about the state of the *relationship* (as with the parent who utilizes guilt feelings to manipulate the child), but about the mental or physical state of the parent herself. High ratings are likely to be given wherever a physically or emotionally ill parent is living in a household, which is not well enough organized by other older members to protect the child from taking the parenting role. (In many households, mental or physical illness on the part of the parent may be looked after by other household members, so that psychological parenting of the sick parent does not become the child's concern.)

(Note: Many or most subjects will rate a "1" on this scale.)

Indices of incompetence, implicit need for care, or role-reversal in childhood:

- Taking care of children seems a bit too much for the parent and *for this reason* it may be left to someone else.
- Parent seems a bit confused or helpless, or a bit of a ditherer. Parent is not a real adult herself.
- Subject's parent complains the children are too much for her, or it is too *hard* to handle them. Implication is again incompetence, rather than rejection or even simply neglect.
- Parent worries that child will get hurt, or is a bit over-protective. Low rating if parent's worrying is just prospective, as, "I wish you wouldn't go rock-climbing", and if parent would actually respond very competently if child actually got hurt. But a high rating if parent would then fall apart herself.
- Subject remembers wanting to protect the parent (higher or lower depending upon whether this was an incident or a general sense, and whether or not the parent welcomed this feeling).
- Subject mentions that the parent was afraid of or unable to stand up to the other parent and hence was weak in the role of protector. Take into consideration only if this is mentioned by the subject.
- Parent was a martyr, a complainer, or a guilt-inducer about or with children.

- Parent accuses child of not wanting the parent around, not loving the parent, not paying enough attention to the parent. Parent needs nearness and attention.
- Subject worries or is worried about hurting the parent's feelings in childhood.
- Child feels guilty about something about the parent; although parent's role in this is not clear (higher rating if it appears that the parent encouraged this feeling).
- Parent uses guilt with child, not to keep child from hurting others, but with reference to hurting the parent herself.
- Child steps in to advise the parent on how to behave as a parent.
- Child is afraid to leave the parent as parent needs the child (rate higher the younger the child is or the more desperate the parent appears; note, if this is the case currently, perhaps it was the case in childhood).
- Child cannot tell the parent her own fears or problems for fear the parent may need care herself. Care for hurt child is too much for the parent to handle.
- Parent clings to child. Parenting is directly demanded.
- Subject states subject felt directly responsible for parent in childhood.
- Subject states she "was her parent's whole life."
- Parent nagged and criticized, as though secretly dependent upon the child's state or appearance.
- Subject's continual aim through childhood was to please her parent.

1. *Parent's psychological or physical well-being was not made a concern to the child*
   The parent may have been loving and strongly supportive, or rejecting, or neglecting, but the parent did not implicitly or explicitly demand psychological concern from the child.
3. *Slight concern about the parent at times, but parent does not need child and is not child's responsibility*
   Perhaps the parent was a little confused by children, or a little disorganized, or a little weak in facing the other parent, and the child might have had to step into the parent's role vis-à-vis the household at times, but *not* into a parental role vis-à-vis the parent. (Example: The child may have had to help the parent with the younger children because the parent was a bit incompetent, but the child did not have to advise the parent on what to do with children!)

   A parent who is a faint concern in a restricted area, but not incompetent, may also be given this rating. The over-protective parent who would be highly competent, responsible, and calm if the child actually got hurt falls here. The child worries a bit about worrying the parent by rock-climbing but knows the parent would be steady and competent if she actually fell. Rate here also if the child felt guilty, worried, or protective about the parent in a single episode, but there is no sign that this was part of a general pattern, and no sign that this feeling was actually encouraged by the parent.

5. *Parent implicitly or explicitly needs attention or care from the child, or child is persuaded to continually attempt to "please" the parent. However, roles are not really reversed between parent and child*
   Concern for the parent is woven into the relationship. Perhaps the parent seems to need the child around her, so that the child feels guilty leaving home or stayed home occasionally for the sake of the parent. Perhaps the parent made clear that the child could hurt her, and used this technique to keep the child in line, or made the child feel guilty at times. (Rate higher if subject really worries about hurting parent, rather than recognizing this as a technique used to manipulate her behavior.) Perhaps the parent's childishness, her chaotic quality, or her lack of parenting ability and general incompetence were strong enough to begin to be a general problem for those around her. Still, for this rating, roles are not really *reversed* between the parent and child.
7. *Beginning of role-reversal*
   The child distinctly began to feel the parent's state, feelings, and protection as a continuing concern. This may have been because of a chaotic household and an unstable parent who implicitly demanded and received care, or because of some deliberate action on the part of the parent. Perhaps the parent felt that the child could not do enough for her, and the child continually wishes to please this parent. Perhaps the child could not tell the parent her own problems, NOT because the parent would be disinterested or angry, but because the parent would actually fall apart in anxiety or chaotic anger herself.
   The balance is beginning to shift, with the child beginning to feel excessively responsible for the parent or the parent's feelings. The child is the parent's "whole life" in some sense, and hence the parent is dependent upon her. Still the parent is competent in some areas.
9. *Role-reversal*
   The parent actively clings to the child and/or the child definitely feels responsible for the care of the parent. The parent may collapse at times, or may collapse whenever there is a problem. The parent may still provide some physical care of the child and even be warm toward the child, but psychologically, the child feels herself to be the responsible and parental member of the dyad.

Present States of Mind with Respect to Attachment:
Coherency, Idealization, Anger, Memory, and Lack of Resolution of Mourning

These scales refer to the mental representation of attachment-related experiences, and/or to the organization of information relevant to attachment. Whereas the preceding five scales assess the adult's inferred experiences of the parents in childhood, the succeeding scales assess the current state of mind with respect to attachment. Some refer to the ease with which information is accessed, some to the apparent distortion that some information has undergone, some to overall organization, and some to feeling. In each case, however, we are dealing with *current* representations of the self in relationship to attachment figures, attachment-related experiences, and attachment-related phenomena.

These scales have been selected out of many possible scales for the mental representation of attachment. They are selected at present for their power to distinguish among individuals whose current state is classified as *autonomous, detached, enmeshed,* or *disorganized-disoriented* with respect to attachment. Individuals classified as autonomous are marked by strong coherency. Individuals classified as detached are often marked by strong idealization of the parents, insistence upon an inability to recall childhood, and little present anger toward the parents. Individuals classified as enmeshed are often incoherent, and/or angry. They seldom insist upon an inability to recall childhood, however, and only one sub-group shows idealization of the parents. Finally, individuals classified in any one of the three groups may be considered disorganized-disoriented through lack of resolution of mourning.

Coherency of Record

This scale attempts to assess the subject's ability to assess her past and its influences coherently, and in a way which makes it understandable without strong efforts of interpretation by the reader. A first measure of coherency is, then, the extent to which the reader finds a unified, yet free-flowing picture of the subject's experiences, feelings, and viewpoints within the interview, such that none of these require the reader to make her own, differing interpretation. In addition, the interview transcript is considered coherent when the subject seems able to easily point to the principle and rationale behind her responses; has thought or else seems ready to think about her past and its influence; and, yet, is also able to examine and "explore the evidence afresh" within the interview itself. In general, the interview is considered coherent when there is a steady and yet developing flow of ideas regarding relationships, events and their influences, and when the reader feels free to record her assessments almost exactly as presented by the subject (i.e., without providing alternative descriptions and interpretations).

In assessing the coherency of the record, look for the way the subject opens up the past, how she focuses on what the interviewer wants to know, and the consistency of her thoughts and feelings about her past with reference to the events, feelings, and related outcomes. Does her overall evaluation and abstract or semantic interpretation of her experiences seem consonant both with the episodes that she recalls and describes and the reader's own interpretation?

N.B. What we are assessing here is coherency of *ideation*, and interference with such coherency. Some speakers use pause markers frequently, as, "We were living in, uh, uh, a small town in Holland." Others stammer, as, "We, we, we were living in Holland." Pause markers and stammering are not important unless patterned so as to interfere with coherency. The scale does not ask for a judgment on the subject's vocabulary or sentence structure but rather considers the interview as a whole, the coherency *between* sentences and paragraphs, the development of ideas, and how they hold together. A single sentence is incoherent only if it is incoherent in terms of ideation.

Look for:

Contradictions

Check the subject's first statement or adjectival summary on relationships to parents against the rest of the information on childhood relationships, separations, rejection, threats, etc. This is a good beginning point in the search for contradictions. For instance, a subject might say "my mother was always there" in the beginning of the interview and later relate that when subject was 18 months, the mother started working 6 days a week, and indicate that her mother ignored her when present. If the subject does not take any note of such contradictions, the contradictions become a mark of incoherency. Contradictions are especially important if the subject is unaware of them and uses them. On the other hand, the subject may recognize and expand upon contradictions. In this case, contradiction becomes much less of a mark of incoherency.

Look especially for three types of contradiction:

- Contradiction between the abstract, generalized, or semantic level of description of attachment figures and experiences, and the episodic level of description.
- Logical contradictions.
- Factual contradictions. Contradictions in the description of the same event or episode, that is, strong contradiction in the "facts" regarding the story being told.

Irrational changes, wordings, and connections within or between sentences

- Strange remarks, or comments that seem out of place. Invasions into speech which interrupt the flow of ideas and whose source or intention is unapparent except through interpretation of themes, conflicts, or unconscious processes personal to the subject.
- Changing standpoints or viewpoints without showing understanding or giving explanation.
- Odd explanations or biases. For example, the subject may state, "I had a good relationship with my father because he was so tall." Or the subject may state, "Rejected? No. There would be no reason why because I always wore yellow." Or the subject may refer to "the mother" or "the father" when she means her own parents.

Irrelevancies

The subject drifts around among ideas or among subjects that are irrelevant or unconnected to the question. The subject tells long stories, which are unrelated to the question, attracts attention to items in the immediate environment, or talks on at great length regarding topics related to the topic only obliquely. The impression given is that the question is unacceptable, so that the answer cannot be sustained and expanded. The subject seems not to be organized in a way that permits her to assess her own experiences and what is being asked about them. Occasionally, the subject may lose track of the question entirely, asking eventually, "What was the question?"

Rapid oscillations of "viewpoint" or "voice"

The subject takes different viewpoints regarding the same phenomena in very rapid succession, often changing viewpoints in mid-sentence. Thus, she states, "It was negative, no, I mean positive," or, "It was horrible, but of course it was right because they were doing what was best," as though correcting or controlling statements through oscillation.

1. *Highly incoherent*
   The subject is so incoherent that the reader is engaged in an intense struggle in attempting to understand and interpret the subject's experiences, feelings, and viewpoints. On close examination of the transcript, the subject may appear irrational.
3. *Incoherent*
   The subject is incoherent to some degree throughout the interview, or there is such contradiction within the interview (e.g., between abstract descriptions and actual memories) that the subject seems not to possess a coherent picture of experiences. Still, the subject does not appear irrational, and the reader can interpret the interview with effort.
5. *Neither coherent nor incoherent*
   Either this subject is coherent for the greater part of the interview but struggles with incoherency over a single issue or for a single period, or there is simply an average degree of coherency throughout the record.
7. *Coherent*
   The transcript has most of the features of coherency described above, but slight incoherencies. Nonetheless, these provide the reader with no more than a little effort of interpretation. The subject does not seem to be in contradiction with herself and her presentation has an easy directedness.
9. *Highly coherent*
   The subject has a steady and developing flow of ideas regarding the attachment-related questions addressed within this interview. The transcript seems in consequence well-organized. However, while her thoughts seem organized, the subject's sentences still seem "fresh" and the subject is in no way pseudo-psychological or pseudo-analytical. The subject seems ready to adapt to new ideas and to experience new insights even while the interview is in progress.

Idealization of the Parent

This scale assesses the discrepancy between the overall viewpoint of the parent taken from the subject's speech at the abstract or semantic level, and the reader's inferences regarding the actual experience of the parent, as based upon other aspects of the transcript. Since the reader has no real knowledge of the real parent, any discrepancies termed idealization come from the transcript itself.

This scale is intended to assess the extent to which the subject retains some image of a "perfect" parent, separated from actual experience. Because the adult interview transcript contains reference both to this "image" and to contradictory thoughts or experiences, the reader is able to develop a score for idealization. The word *idealization* refers to the fact that the parent is idealized, or turned into an *idea* (cf. Bishop Berkeley), such that semantic storage of the parent is as "good" or "entirely normal," where episodic memories may be completely unsupportive of this picture.

This scale is not intended to assess every type of distortion in the subject's representation of the parent. High scores on this scale are given to individuals who, for example, describe the parent and the relationship as "fine" or "excellent" but whose memories seem entirely memories of rejection. The scale is not intended to be used for parents who say, in a single brief paragraph or sentence, "The relationship was negative – no, maybe it was positive"; "He was awful to do that to me, but I'm thankful and grateful for it because it was for the best"; "She was terrific – no, actually, I've wound up with a lot of problems." These subjects express contradictory or confused "images" of the parent, but the images appear almost simultaneously or else in rapid sequence.

In rating a subject for idealization of the parent, it is useful to take an especially close look at (a) the subject's first description of the parent; (b) any out-of-context praise of parents, for example, "excellent, wonderful parents"; (c) the subject's response to the rejection question – whether it stands up realistically against the "upset and run to" question, or against other anecdotes, especially ones on conflict and separation experiences. The subject is considered to idealize the parent more where praise of the parent is unqualified, and where there is no concrete or specific supporting evidence. There may be an odd choice of words, such as, "She was an *excellent* mother," in answer to, "How would you describe your relationship with your mother?" There may be a lack of anything personal in the way in which the subject describes what the parent did.

Note: The *distance* between the image of the parent and inferred experience is important. The individual who recalls abuse, but regards the parent as "pretty supportive and normal" rather than "perfect" is considered strongly idealizing – perhaps as strongly idealizing as the individual who simply can recall nothing positive while describing the parent as excellent, wonderful, or perfect.

1. *No idealization*

   The subject may feel her parent was the best she could have possibly had, but she is aware of the ups and downs in the relationship, and anecdotes are entirely supportive of this picture.

3. *Slight idealization of parent*
   There is some tendency to distance a picture of a "good and supportive" parent from description of real feelings, relationships, or episodes, but it is entirely within a range that is expectable.
5. *Moderate idealization of the parent*
   There is a distinct distance between the image of the parent and descriptions, memories, or feelings, such that the reader is fully aware of a difference. Still, the idealization of the parent is incomplete, and the subject seems aware of difficulties even though these remain unintegrated.
7. *Idealization of the parent*
   There is an unmistakable lack of unity between the description of the parent and the reader's estimate of probable experience. There is a striking splitting within the interview between descriptions of the parent as "normal" or "fine" or "supportive" and the failure to access memories of real support, and/or actual memories of lack of support or cruelty to self or others. By the readers best estimate, the parent was not loving or was actively rejecting – but the subject consistently insists upon the impression of "a fine relationship." Still, as compared to the subject rated a 9, this subject has occasional access to negative memories or experiences (which are not considered to reflect upon the parent).
9. *Strong idealization of the parent*
   In the reader's assessment, the parent was not loving and may have had actively negative qualities such as strong rejection. The subject's portrait of the parent is nonetheless consistently either positive or innocuous. There is no real criticism, and any difficulties, which can be inferred from close reading of the interview, are not attributed to the parent. The parent is presumed to have had no negative effects; to have been normal, fine, excellent, or acceptable in terms of parenting. The lack of unity in the portrait of the parent is unmistakable. Either the parent is portrayed as perfect without supporting evidence, or evidence of cruelty or coldness is given while the parent is portrayed as entirely normal.

Anger Expressed Toward Parent Now

This scale rates the extent to which the subject expresses anger toward the parent within the interview. The anger is evident in speech, that is, is "conscious" in the common sense. The reader's sense of the subject's anger does not rely upon dynamic interpretations of repressed or unexpressed emotions; repressed, unexpressed anger is not being rated. Some readers might infer that a subject who stated, "My mother is a very, very wonderful person – I've never had cause to question anything she did" was more angry with the parent than a subject who stated, "My mother is a mean old witch." On this scale, however, the first sentence would not be taken into account, since there is no expressed anger. The second sentence would be taken into account.

The anger rated here can appear either in discussions of the past or in response to queries regarding the present relationship. The anger rated in this scale is clearly connected to the parent, but may or may not be shown to the parent in real life. The following would be indices of "anger toward the parent now":

- "Why she would do things like that to me, God only knows."
- "She had a LOT of problems."
- "She still hasn't got the sense she was born with."
- "He won't recognize me as an independent person – never has, never will."

Sentences communicating comparable content, but without indices of current anger are:

- "I still have a hard time understanding what made her do that."
- "My mother was probably experiencing her own difficulties at the time."
- "It's regretful, but she still isn't a person you could call either mature or sensible."

  "I don't think he's developed much further in terms of seeing me as independent."

1. *No direct expression of anger*
3. *Slight annoyance*
   Subject is a bit annoyed with the parent (in interview or in real life).
5. *Anger*
   Anger is currently sufficient that there are mounting tensions or flare-ups, or the subject seems a bit mad at the moment, but there is no evidence that anger toward the parent has become a theme in subject's life.
7. *Thematic anger*
   Anger toward the parent is a theme in the interview or within the subject's life, but subject can describe other aspects of the relationship or has still some relationship to parent.
9. *Direct anger*
   It is almost impossible for the subject to interact calmly with the parent in real life, and/or to describe the parent or relationship to the parent during the interview beyond aspects of anger.

Frequency and Strength of Insistence Upon Inability to Recall Childhood

In order to begin rating this variable, it is necessary to have examined and rated a range of transcripts. The ideal topic of the scale would of course be the subject's actual inability to recall childhood; this, however, cannot be known or rated. What we attempt to rate and scale here is, therefore, instead the subject's frequency and strength of insistence upon an inability to recall childhood. Once the range is established, this can be estimated.

1. *No insistence upon inability to recall childhood.*
3. *Infrequent or slight insistence upon inability to recall childhood.*
5. *Some insistence upon inability to recall childhood.*
7. *Frequent or strong insistence upon inability to recall childhood.*
9. *Very frequent or very strong insistence upon inability to recall childhood.*

5 Relationship Representation in Child–Parent Discourse

Instructions for Classifying Seven Central Patterns

Amy Strage and Mary Main

This is a set of instructions for identifying dyadic attachment organization through a study of discourse transcripts obtained within a relatively uncontrolled laboratory setting. The system was developed by using knowledge of individual differences in attachment organization as seen in the Ainsworth Strange Situation (Ainsworth et al., 1978; Main & Solomon, 1986; Main & Hesse, 1990), the Clown Session (Main & Weston, 1981), and analyses of the Adult Attachment Interview to develop an understanding of the type of organization, which dyads of different types experience, preserve, or are attempting to preserve. Using our original Berkeley follow-up study sample (described in Main et al., 1985), we were able to identify three of the four major types of infant attachment organization (A, B, D) from a study of speech transcripts alone (Strage & Main, 1985). Hit-rates for the three major groups for both mother–child and father–child dyads were above 80%: Hit-rates for sub-groups were lower but still significant. Too few group C dyads were available to develop a discourse pattern with this first sample. However, with transcripts loaned from other investigators, we are now mid-way to developing discourse equivalencies for this fourth major attachment pattern.

Procedure

Parents and children were brought to our laboratory for a series of individual and family assessments involving attachment. Following a brief period in which the child was introduced to the laboratory playroom (in which she would be continually video-taped) while the parents spoke with the interviewers in the project office, the parents joined the child in the playroom to watch a movie of a child undergoing a major separation from parents (see George, 1984). Mothers and fathers then went to separate offices for the Adult Attachment Interview assessment, while the child remained in the laboratory playroom doing drawings, responding to questions regarding what children feel and do about separations (Kaplan, 1987), and finally engaging in free, undirected play involving a sandbox and numerous small figures and toys.

When the parents returned to the room at the end of the session, the child had been in the laboratory for a total of approximately 2 hours. Reunions

DOI: 10.4324/9781003569978-5

were balanced so that mother (father) returned first in half the cases, while father (mother) returned 3 minutes later. Beyond this, we made no effort to control these reunion episodes. Parents were simply told that the session was over; the other parent would arrive shortly; and that the interviewers would be bringing forms to the parents for final signature. The examiner remained in the room throughout the reunion episode.

We offer a historical rather than a prescriptive view of this much of our procedure because it is certainly possible that a more controlled procedure could produce still sharper relationship distinctions. The overloaded cast of characters provided by our relatively uncontrolled situation seemed, however, to reduce self-consciousness, and permitted adults who did not want to address the child to instead address the examiner or the other parent (while children too could choose to address someone other than the returning parent).

It is possible, too, that we heightened opportunity for observing relationship organization through stressing themes of attachment and separation for both child and parent not long before reunion. For the adult in particular, themes of attachment must have been prominent. As noted above, the parents in the Berkeley follow-up study entered the playroom immediately following an intensive interview focused upon their own attachment histories and experiences of separation or loss of attachment figures through death.

Transcription of Discourse for the Reunion Episode

Reunions with each parent lasted approximately 3 minutes. Transcripts of all discourse occurring during the reunion episode were made directly from video-tapes of the full reunion episode. Transcripts included the speech of the examiner as well as the child and parent. When the second parent entered the room, the first parent was, of course, present and remained so. However, although transcription of the speech of the first parent continued, the child–parent reunion discourse with the first parent was considered completed; transcription for the second parent now began.

Transcripts included speech dysfluencies (false starts, pause markers, etc.); rough estimates of the duration of pauses within speech or between speakers lasting more than 1 second; and marks for speaker overlap. There seems to us to be little doubt that, with the use of vocalic cues included, discourse equivalencies to early attachment organization would be even more sharply defined. Our interest was, however, in the representational rather than the emotional aspects of speech. We therefore removed all cues to emotional tone or status, and failed to record concomitant non-verbal behavior. The transcripts were devoid of information regarding prosody and intonation. Words were recorded as written speech. Once transcripts had been completed, mother–child and father–child transcripts were divided and given to a psycholinguist who was not only blind to early attachment classifications but also had never seen the dyads in any context beyond these particular transcripts.

Our presentation of rules for the identification of each category is accompanied by excerpts from transcripts from the Berkeley sample. As noted previously, 80% (51) of the 64 Berkeley transcripts were identified correctly for major category, and 67% (43) were identified correctly as fitting into one of the full seven (A1, A2, B1, B2, B3, B4, D) categories. The excerpts, which we present, are taken from transcripts which had been correctly identified by the judge.

In reading the transcripts, it will be helpful for the reader to be informed that, at the beginning of the session (and when the parents were last in the room), the child's sandbox had been hidden, and appeared as simply a table. In addition, as noted earlier, children were usually engaged in sandbox play when the parents entered the room.

Much conversation took place between the examiner and the parents, or the child and the other parent. Here we largely excerpt only those portions of conversation taking place between the child and the parent with whom she had been secure in infancy. The ellipsis to the left margin indicates that portions of discourse (often including the examiner or the second parent) have been eliminated. Throughout this chapter, where the child's real name is used, we have substituted Adam or Eve.

No insecure-resistant coding scheme was developed due to too few dyads in the recall sample.

Discourse Classifications

There are three major discourse classifications in our system – fluent, restricted, and dysfluent – reflecting the secure, insecure-avoidant, and disorganized/disoriented infant attachment categories, respectively. In addition, we distinguish between the discourse structures of the two insecure-avoidant (A1 vs. A2) and the four secure (B1, B2, B3, and B4) sub-groups of attachment organizations identified in the Ainsworth Strange Situation. The primary dimensions under consideration are:

1. *The fluidity of the dialogue.* This we identify as the mechanical aspects of the dialogue, such as whether questions were answered, and how promptly; where pauses in the verbal interchanges occur; where and whether interruptions and orderly exchange of the floor (turn-taking) occur; when speakers stumble over words or made false starts.
2. *The focus of the discourse.* The ways in which objects and the partners or other individuals in the room are talked about; whether topics of conversation are restricted or free to shift.
3. *The dialectics of the discourse.* This refers to the dynamic balance of the conversation, such as whether topics introduced by one speaker are taken up and elaborated on by the other; or quickly dismissed; or superseded by the introduction of another topic; whether partners implicitly offer "turns" to one another, advancing the dialectic; or whether one partner consistently leads the flow of the conversation, while the second Is passive in response.

Fluent Discourse

As infants, children securely attached to mother have had both physical and psychological access to her throughout their infancy. In the home situation, as compared to other mothers, the mothers of Group B infants are described by Ainsworth as "sensitive to the signals and communications of their infants" (Ainsworth et al., 1971), a finding which has been replicated several times (see Bretherton (1985) for a summary). This given, we would expect to observe what we have defined as fluidity of discourse, as well as optimal dialectical properties, in these children, which in fact we do.

At the beginning of the Strange Situation, Group B infants focus their attention upon toys and novel objects in the environment; following one or two separations from the parent, they make clear their desire to re-establish proximity, contact, or interaction. For the prototypical, "very secure" B3 infant, the return of the parent permits the child to settle and eventually return to play. The same easy alternation between attention to objects and attention to the attachment figure has been observed in the home situation (Ainsworth et al., 1971). In terms of topics, then, we would expect little or no restriction.

Group B and Group B3

Child–parent discourse is categorized as *fluent* when it has the characteristics of good dialogue. The following parameters characterize Group B discourse in general, and characterize the discourse of the very secure B3 dyads particularly.

1. There are few or no ignored conversational overtures by parent or child.
2. There are no long pauses except between topics, or after a completed cycle of turn exchanges.
3. Few rhetorical questions, test questions, or yes/no answer questions from either party. Questions the partners ask of one another appear to be genuine information-seeking, and leave open the partner's opportunity to expand or elaborate in response.
4. Topics do not appear to be restricted to a particular focus, and may shift focus or be elaborated.
5. Neither partner is dysfluent or disorganized in speech.
6. Both parties may persist in moving topics forward.

Beyond the above six parameters, it is difficult to characterize the discourse of B3 dyads. This is because, as opposed to discourse seen in the less secure dyads, no particular rules prevail. Thus, the discourse of the B3 dyad is determined by the fact that (a) it is neither restricted nor dysfluent; (b) it fits, in general terms, to the characteristics as defined above and (c) it cannot be further identified through any of the rules characterizing the

B1, B2, or B4 dyads. This means that the discourse of the B3 dyad may be extensive or brief; the child's apparent attitude to the parent may be cooperative or warmly sassy; the partners may appear interested in conversation with one another or, on the other hand, engaged in non-verbal activities apart or together.

In Figures 5.1a–5.1d, we provide excerpts from several B3 transcripts.

Father: What'd you do?
Child: Played with sand.
Father: Why, I didn't even know you had sand in this deal. How'd ya, did you put it there?
Child: No, she did.
Father: I didn't even know that. I should have guessed, I guess, that there was a sandbox.
Child: It was under there.
. . .
Father: Hey, Eve.
Child: What?
Father: You know something? You know how your brothers have all those army guys like this?
Child: Yeah.
Father: When I was growing up I didn't have army guys, I had guys like this . . . I betcha these are really old.
Child: I betcha they aren't.

Figure 5.1a B3 Discourse

Father: What are, what, what are you making there, Adam?*
Child: Sandcastle.
Father: Sandcastle?
Child: Yeah.
Father: That's a lot of fun.
Child: Wanna help?
Father: Yeah, I'll help out there.
. . .
Father: A castle is a house. You know what a castle is, Adam?
Child: What?
Father: What's a castle? You know what a castle is?
Child: This looks like a mountain to me. What about to you?
. . .
Father: I was gonna ask you. Do you know what a, what a, what a castle is?
Child: No.

Figure 5.1b B3 Discourse

Father: A castle is a house that a king lives in.
Child: Does a king live, um, does a king live in it, does it?
Father: A king lives in a castle, yes . . . And nowadays, there're not too many kings around. Not in this country.
Child: Why?
Father: well . . .
Child: There's not too many, right?
Father: Not in this country, there aren't any kings.
Child: But there's queens.
Father: No, there's no queens either.
Child: Where is there kings and queens? . . . What about in Tahoe?

* This parent's speech is unusually dysfluent for the B3 category. Interestingly, on the basis of the child's Strange Situation behavior as an infant, both B4 and D categories had been considered as alternatives.

Figure 5.1b (Continued)

Mother: Hi. Did you think we were lost?
Child: What?
Mother: Did you think we were lost?
Child: No.
Mother: You're having fun, huh? Having fun. May I feel it?
Child: Yeah.
Mother: Oooo . . . doesn't that feel good . . . That's like the one you had a nursery school, isn't it? But they used cornmeal.
Child: Put your hand right here, mommy. Put your hand right here. Mommy, put your hand right here. Put your hand right here, Mom.
. . .
Mother: So, have you just been playing in the sand, or what?
Child: We've been playing in the sand, and looking at pictures.
Mother: Really?
Child: And.
Mother: What?
Child: (giggles).
Mother: Secrets, huh? Okay.
. . .
Mother: Oooo, what kind is that?
Child: A red one.
Mother: But what is it? Do you have any idea what it might be?
Child: An ambulance.

Figure 5.1c B3 Discourse

Child: Awww.
Mother: Aw, I'm back. Hey, that's sand. That's what was under there. I didn't know that.
Child: Mmm.
Mother: Tired yet?
Child: No.
Mother: That what I told her (the interviewer). You were a night-owl.
Child: See, this is a trap-door.
Mother: Oh. What happens if it's – oh, and they end up in the prison down there?
Child: Yeah. Yep.
Mother: Put something in and show me.
Child: Okay. See. Here's one.

Figure 5.1d B3 Discourse

Sub-Group B1

As infants seen in the Ainsworth Strange Situation, children in the B1 sub-group are identified on reunion for substituting an enthusiastic greeting, and initiations of interaction across a distance (often vocal interchanges), for the proximity and contact-seeking of other secure infants. These children are unlikely to show distress upon separation, focusing instead upon the toys or stranger.

Observed in the Clown Session, the parents of the B1 infants show much delight in the infant, combined with some aversion to physical contact. Analysis of the parent's own attachment history, and present state of mind with respect of attachment as seen in the Adult Attachment Interview shows that the parents can be described as valuing attachment, but as often actively setting aside their own attachment histories or relationships. The adult is characteristically described as having re-evaluated and re-directed his or her life following somewhat harsh experiences of early relationships. The adult shares some characteristics with adults in the dismissing category.

Given this much information regarding this dyad outside of the speech context, we would expect discourse for these dyads to be largely fluent, to place emphasis upon language and/or the types of interaction made especially available through language, and to bear some resemblance to restricted discourse patterns. This is in fact what is found.

Fluent dyads are placed in the B1 sub-category when discourse has all or most of the following features:

1. Topics largely restricted to the here-and-now, with little direct reference to personal states or to relationship;
2. Fluid dialogue with much speech and elaboration on the part of both partners;

3. Specifiable, readily answerable questions, for example, what are you doing/making, but not rhetorical or test questions;
4. Logical explanations or games involving logic or violations of logic, puns, metaphors, or play on words.

Excerpts taken from B1 transcripts are exhibited in Figures 5.2a–5.2d.

Father: Hello.
Child: I wanna stay here.
Father: (Laughs).
Child: I'm not going.
Father: No. Really?
Child: Yeah.
Father: We can come back tomorrow and get you?
Child: Yeah. No.
Father: The day after tomorrow?
Child: Next week. Two weeks.
Father: Two weeks? Oh, that would be nice, huh?
Child: Two weeks.
Father: You know where the bathroom is and everything and where the food is?
Child: No, they're going to tell us.

Figure 5.2a B1 Discourse

Child: Hi . . . Hi. Time to go?
Father: I don't know. They asked me to come in here. What are you doing?
Child: Uh, nothing really, I'm just playing. That's all I'm doing.
Father: What are you playing?
Child: The castle and all that stuff.
Father: What did you do while I was gone?
Child: A lot of stuff.
Father: What? Tell me.
Child: Umm. I'll show you the picture that I . . .
Father: . . . oh yeah, I want to see pictures.
Child: Here's one. Here's our family in a rowboat. with some clouds and the sun . . .
Father: Who's here? Tell me everybody.
Child: Okay, I'll tell you everybody. That's you rowing the boat.
Father: How come I have to row?
Child: (Laughs). You're the strongest.
Father: Oh, okay.

Figure 5.2b B1 Discourse

Father: How come Lori's in the middle?
Child: Cuz she's safer with you two guys.
Father: You're right . . . Well, why didn't you put Annette on the inside too, then? You know she's littler than you. You stuck her way out there on the end, you know.
Child: I know. She's supposed to be there.
Father: Is she? Why?
Child: That's where the seatbelts are.
Father: Oh, okay. These are seatbelts?

Figure 5.2b (Continued)

Child: Hi, Dad.
Father: Hi, Adam.
Child: I got my shoes and socks off, so I can go in there.
Father: You sure do. Have you been having a good time?
Child: Yep.
Father: You haven't been spreading sand all over the place, have you?
. . .
Child: This is a giant sea monster.
Father: Mm. Looks like cousin Fred, doesn't he?

Figure 5.2c B1 Discourse

Father: Hi, kid.
One-and-one-third-second pause
Child: Hi.
Father: What are you building here, huh?
Child: Playing.
Father: What? What are you–
Child: Playing.
Father: Well, what do you build? Something there, huh?
Child: Playing. Just playing, that's all.
Father: Are they going to fall, those houses? You build the tower of Babel, huh? (Laughs).
A 7-second pause
Father: So did you have fun, Adam?
Child: Yep.
Father: You want me to play with you? Can I play too?
Child: Yeah.
Father: See if I can put this up – like that, you see.
Child: Wait. You have to stick it in hard.

Figure 5.2d B1 Discourse

Father: okay, not too hard, not too hard.
Child: All the way to the ground.
Father: Why?
Child: You have to stick it that far so it doesn't fall down.
Father: Okay. Now we're going to put it on top of each other. I want a tall tower.
Child: No.
. . .
Child: No, leave it. It protects from dinosaurs.

Figure 5.2d (Continued)

Sub-Group B2

In the Ainsworth Strange Situation, secure infants are placed in the B2 sub-category when they show some avoidance of the parent in the first reunion episode, but actively seek to achieve proximity and contact with the parent during the second reunion. Essentially, then, infants are classified as B2 within the Strange Situation when they resemble avoidant infants at first, then behavior as secure infants.

Observed in the home situation (Ainsworth et al., 1971), the parents of B2 infants are found moderately sensitive, although they may be inconsistent in their sensitivity (sometimes sensitive, sometimes insensitive) rather than continually moderate. In the Adult Attachment Interview, adults who seem essentially secure but also have some of the characteristics of the dismissing adult group are placed in this category.

Given these characteristics as observed outside of the discourse context, we would expect discourse which fits most of the criteria for *fluent* discourse, but which shows also some resemblance to transcripts classified as *restricted.* Fluent dyads are placed in the B2 category when they show some or all of the following features:

1. Resemblances to the behavior of restricted dyads are as follows:
   a. The partners may be somewhat perfunctory in asking questions or answering them.
   b. Pauses between conversational turns are longer than for B3 dyads.
   c. The focus of the conversation may be (but is not necessarily) more related to objects and activities than is the case for B3 dyads.
   d. The parent may initiate conversation with an exaggerated exclamation, which does not provide opportunity for turn-taking by the partner, then add a comment or further question which provides an opening, for example, "Wow! That's a great truck!", followed shortly by, "How long have you been playing with it?".
   e. As in some of the restricted dyads, much of the adult's speech may be directed to the examiner, or apparently directed to the child but with the examiner clearly equally directly in focus.

2. Nonetheless, the discourse is essentially fluent. Interestingly, as in the case of the infant's initially avoidant, then "secure" Strange Situation behavior, a B2 discourse often begins with some restriction, and then becomes more fluent.

Figures 5.3a–5.3c provide excerpts from several B2 transcripts.

Mother: Wow! Look at that, Adam. Is that ever neat!
One-and-one-half-second pause
Mother: Did (examiner) do all that? Is that your name?
Examiner: Yeah.
Mother: Yeah.
Child: No.
Mother: Huh? No? I bet she did.
Child: No.
Mother: No? Did you do most of it?
Child: I did all of it.
Mother: All of it? I love it. I just love it.
One-and-four-tenths-second pause
Child: The dinosaurs are over there.
Mother: Yeah. I see that. Yeah, and you got the farm and the animals and the town. That's really great. We're gonna have to get your sandbox filled back up again this summer. It's hard to find good, the right kind of sand.
Examiner: Yeah.
Mother: They want to deliver it in big tons or . . . or if you buy little, our sandbox is, you know, quite a bit bigger than this, so one or two bags won't do it if you buy the little bags.

Figure 5.3a B2 Discourse

Child: Hi, Dad.
Father: Hi, Adam. How are you?
Child: What are you doing?
Father: I came to see what you're doing. I'm done.
Child: What about Mom?
Father: I don't know where Mom is.
Child: I guess she's done.
Father: That's pretty neat, huh?
Child: Uh huh.
. . .
Child: I can make, I make, I can make some nice smooth land.

Figure 5.3b B2 Discourse

Father: Oh, yeah.
Six-second pause
Father: It's like down at the beach.
Two-second pause
Child: Yeah.
Ten-second pause
Child: I wonder what Mom's doing now?
Father: She's probably just finishing up. I think I hear her coming.
Six-second pause
Father: You getting tired?

Figure 5.3b (Continued)

Six conversational turns take place before mother or child speak to one another

Child: Mommy, I'm sweaty as a pig.
Mother: A pig? How do you know how a pig sweats?
Two-second pause
Mother: I want to see – I want to see what you made.
Can I just move this?
Child: Mommy, look what I made. Look what, look what I made.
Mother: Hey, that's neat. What is it?
One-and-one-half-second pause
Child: It's me. That could be a chipmunk, a squirrel.
Mother: Talk about it. What is it? Tell me more.

Figure 5.3c B2 Discourse

Sub-Group B4

In the Ainsworth Strange Situation, an infant is judged to fall in the B4 sub-category when it focuses more upon the parent than the toys throughout the situation; shows more distress upon separation than a B3 infant; and following the second separation seems less interested in a return to play with toys than in maintaining proximity and contact with the mother. There are obvious resemblances to the insecure-resistant Group C infant behaviors here, but the B4 infant is not so angry, and is able eventually to be settled. There are also some resemblances to Group D, the disorganized/disoriented infants, in that infants judged B4 sometimes show episodes of disorganization. If they do, however, they differ from infants ultimately placed in category D in that they follow these apparent episodes of distress with approaches to the attachment figure.

In the Adult Attachment Interview, Group B4 parents are identified as being somewhat dependent, sentimental, or faintly incoherent in their descriptions and understanding of their past experiences. These experiences, as they describe them, are various: from backgrounds in which some over-protection seems a feature, to background in which trauma in the form of death, loss, or even abuse was featured. Despite some incoherency in the description of events, a strong sense of self often emerges in these interviews.

This given, we would expect some resemblance in the B4 transcripts to the dysfluent (D) transcripts, and this is indeed what we find. An interesting reversal can be seen between the impression given by the Strange Situation assessment – that is, that it is the infant who is particularly dependent – and the impression given by the transcript, which is that the dependency is now the property of the parent, who to some extent is conversationally supported by the child.

Fluent dyads are placed in the B4 sub-category when they meet some or all of the following criteria:

1. Child rather than parent provides conversational scaffolding.
2. A number of empty turns are filled with exclamation or apology.
3. One partner may move to a conversational tangent for some period of time.
4. The focus or topic of the discourse is sometimes more personal, or relationship-focused, than is the case with B3 dyads.
5. Some affirmation-seeking tag-end questions are used by the parent.

Excerpts from several B4 transcripts are presented in Figures 5.4a–5.4c.

Mother: Hello.
Child: Mom, is it time to go?
Mother: In a little bit. What are you doing?
Child: What does it look like I'm doing?
Mother: Wow, it looks like you're making a corral. That's great.
(Discussion follows, largely between father and child, regarding a horse named Kanga which the family used to have.)
Mother: This looks kind of like Kanga.
Child: No, it doesn't.
Mother: Sorry (giggles).
Child: Kanga has a white tush.
Mother: I'm sorry (giggles).
Child: And needs to be pregnant.
. . .
Mother: Kanga was built more like this horse.
Child: Yeah. No. I'll show you what Kanga's built like.
Mother: Like what (giggles).
Child: Like that.

Figure 5.4a B4 Discourse

Mother: Like a pig, eh. I was afraid you'd hit me if I said Kanga looked like a pig.

. . .

Mother: That's a huge corral. It's a long one. The horse can run a long way in that corral, Start at this end and then run clear down to the other end.
Child: Mom, this is not going to be exactly a corral.
Mother: Oh, it's not?

Figure 5.4a (Continued)

Child: Mom.
Mother: Hello.
Child: Mom, you know what the surprise is?
Mother: What? Hey!
Child: We made a giant sandcastle. You know what I wish I could keep? I wish I could keep this. You know why?
Mother: Why?
Child: I, I, I, used to have one of these but I don't.
Mother: Sure ya did. yeah. You probably, uh, used it so much it wore out or something.

. . .

Mother: Wow, you got to use a lot of neat things, didn't you, Adam? Did you use all of this stuff?
Child: Yeah.
Mother: Yeah.
Child: Except for, for, the things that are in here. I used some dinosaurs and I used that –
Mother: Yeah.
Child: –and I used that and I used–
Mother: Yeah.
Child: –that.
Mother: That's neat.
Child: Some, some monsters came down on the castle.
Mother: Yeah?

Figure 5.4b B4 Discourse

Mother: Hi, honey. What ya doing?
Child: Building sand.
Mother: Oh, they have some car caddies like we have at home.
Child: Well, yeah, only they come with sand and toys.
Mother: Oh, they put toys in them instead. Listen, I brought your, what do you call it, Mr. Sandkin?

Figure 5.4c B4 Discourse

Child: You, yeah, my Mr. Sandmachen.
Mother: Sandmachen.
Child: Is it, is it dry?
Mother: No. It's that kind of day that doesn't dry out, I don't think.
. . .
Mother: So did you have a good time, honey?
Child: Yeah. I'm gonna make a sa, um, a sandcastle out of this.
Mother: Ahh.
Child: Okay, mom?
Mother: Mmm hmm.
Child: Okay?
Mother: Sure.
Child: And I'm gonna take a lot of sand make it up now.
Nine-second pause
Mother: Did Dad come by yet?
One-and-one-half-second pause
Mother: Huh?
Child: I didn't see him.
Mother: No? Well, I guess he didn't come by then.

Figure 5.4c (Continued)

Restricted Discourse

In the Ainsworth Strange Situation, the infant is judged insecure-avoidant (Group A) if she shows little or no distress during the parent's absence; actively avoids and ignores the parent upon reunion; and spends the majority of the situation occupied with the toys. Home observations of these infants in Baltimore show active rejection of attachment behavior by the infant's mother (Ainsworth et al., 1971), and, in American samples, a specific aversion on the part of the mother to physical contact (Main & Stadtman, 1981). Adult Attachment Interviews conducted with the parents of insecure-avoidant infants show that the parents are largely dismissing of attachment and the likelihood of the influence of attachment-related experiences upon feeling or personality.

Given this description of the Group A dyad, it is not difficult to imagine the characteristics of the discourse. It is minimal, impersonal, and rhetorical. More specifically, discourse has most or all of the following features:

1. Parent may speak with examiner rather than child.
2. Frequent pauses between adult and child conversational turns.
3. Topic elaboration is limited in quantity and quality, that is, topic is restricted to an impersonal perspective and/or inanimate objects or activities with objects.
4. The parent's questions tend to be rhetorical questions, yes/no answer questions, or test questions.

5. Empty turns by parent.
6. Parent is distinctly in control of the conversation.
7. If the child makes anomalous or tangential overtures or utterances, the parent is unresponsive.
8. Even when addressing the child, the parent's remarks may be implicitly for the benefit of the examiner.

Sub-Group A1

In infancy, these are the most extremely avoidant of infants. They do not show distress during the parent's absence, or even when left entirely alone. Upon reunion, they usually do not show even the slight anger or delayed faint proximity-seeking of the A2 infants. In the Adult Attachment Interview, parents of the A1 infants are often either actively disparaging of attachment figures and feelings, or claim an inability to recall childhood. Our review of discourse transcripts of these dyads shows the general characteristics of the restricted dyad, but in addition:

1. Very long pauses between turns, or even;
2. No parent–child greeting at all and no conversation throughout the reunion.

Of eight A1 dyads available within our Berkeley sample, two were completely silent with respect to one another on reunion (this did not occur in any of the other 62 dyads within the sample). In one case, the mother and examiner talked throughout the episode, but mother and child did not once address each other. In the other case, a father–child reunion, child and mother, mother and father, and child and examiner spoke, but neither child nor father spoke to one another.

Figures 5.5a and 5.5b present excerpts from the discourse of two other A1 dyads.

Mother: Hello.
Child: Look-it.
Mother: What did you do?
One-and-one-half-second pause
Mother: What is that?
Child: It's a space house.
Mother: It's a space house?
Child: Yeah.
Mother: Mmm.

Mother and child do not speak for the remainder of the reunion.

Figure 5.5a A1 Discourse

Father: Hi. There's a sandbox!
Father: How ya doing?
Father: How ya doing?
Child: (Giggles).
Father: Can I play? No.
Child: (Giggles).
Father: Have you seen mother?
Child: No.
Father: No?
(*Father and examiner discuss sandbox*).
Father: We don't have one anymore, do we?
Child: No.
Father: We broke it.
. . .
Father: Has this lady been bothering you?
Child: No.
Father: No. Okay.

Figure 5.5b A1 Discourse

Sub-Group A2

As noted above, infants judged A2 rather than A1 in terms of Strange Situation behavior show more feeling and more proximity-seeking. They may cry when left completely alone in the room; approach the mother very late in the second reunion episode; and show some subtle anger toward the mother when picked up. In the Adult Attachment Interview, the parents of these infants have greater access to attachment-related feelings and memories than the parents of A1 infants, including memories of rejection by parents, but restrict their sense of the effect of these experiences and memories by statements to the effect that these experiences have not affected the self.

This given, it is not surprising that there is a fairly sharp distinction between A2 and A1 discourse. Whereas A1 discourse is unlikely to be confused with B discourse, there is a distinct resemblance between the discourse of A2 and of B2 dyads. The A2 transcript meets most of the general descriptors for restricted discourse, but in addition:

1. The parent may greet the child with empty exclamations which are intended to be positive, but which in effect do not pass or offer the child a response.
2. The parent may indicate interest in the child's activities, but through questions to which it is difficult to formulate a response.
3. As compared to A1 discourse, there is much more conversation.

Figures 5.6a–5.6c give several examples of A2 discourse transcripts. Note that the child typically makes very terse, or even rejecting replies, but that occasionally by the very end of the reunion somewhat more fluent discourse occurs (see Figure 5.6c).

Mother: Wow!
Mother: So, what have you been up to, Adam?
Child: Just draw a picture.
Mother: What'd you draw a picture of?
Child: You have to see it. I can't show you.
. . .
Mother: Is that, what's that top picture? Is that our house?
Child: Uh hum.
Mother: It sure is. You know how I knew it was our house, Adam?
Child: How?
Mother: Because of the swimming pool. Ah hoo . . . ooo, and the orchard.
Mother: I love it. And that's our truck.
(Mother talks about house to examiner for an extended period).
. . .
Mother: Oh Adam, I like that.
Four-and-one-half-second pause
Mother: You even got the right number of wheels on the truck. I was just counting.

Figure 5.6a A2 Discourse

Father: Ahhh, Adam! What've ya been doing? (*One-second pause*). Wondering where the heck I was, right?
Father: What? Did you make all this?
Child: Uh huh.
Father: Oh my God, can I hear about it?
Child: I don't know what to say.
Father: I mean, my God, look at all that.
A 1-second pause
Father: Now, this is a neat thing. You know that?
A 1-second pause
Father: You know, we gotta fix your sandbox up at home?
A 3-second pause
Father: You know that, this is not a bad idea. Would this be a better way to have a sandbox, or do you like the one you can actually be in, too?

Figure 5.6b A2 Discourse

Mother: Hi.
Child: Hi.
Mother: How ya doing?
Child: Fine.
Mother: Hey, look at that! There was sand under there.
Child: Mommy, look it.
Mother: I bet ya they would like to clobber you.
Child: Laughs.
Mother: Adam, don't make (the examiner) work so hard.
Child: Laughs.
A 5-second pause
Mother talks extensively with examiner
Mother: Are you spoiled having somebody to play with for so long?
Child: No.
Mother: Oh well, right.
Mother and examiner talk until end of episode
Child: Hey mommy. Four people had the same lunchbox at school.
Mother: Four? today?
Child: Yeah. That's mine. Timothy had one, uh, Nancy had one, and Cliff had one.
Mother: Well, its a good thing I put your name on it.
Child: Yeah.
Mother: Mm hmm.
Child: They all had names on em.
Mother: Good. Their mothers are smart.

Figure 5.6c A2 Discourse

Mother: Hello, sandbox people.
Mother and father talk.
Mother: What are you doing, Eve?
A 1-second pause
Mother: Is this fun?
Child: Uhm. Yeah, this house is on fire.
Mother: Um, oh my goodness. What's happening?
A 1-second pause
Child: (low mumble).
. . .
Mother: Did you set this up or was it like this?
Child: I set this up.
Mother: The whole thing? All these people in here? Oh my goodness. Who's this?

Figure 5.6d A2 Discourse

Child: (low mumble).
Mother: What are they doing?
Child: Riding horses.
Mother: Does it look like fun? Oh, I like the hats.
A 1-second pause
Mother: Did you put the hats on them?
Child: *Nods.*
A 5-second pause
Mother: Are these castle people? Oh, those are playmobiles.
Child: Yeah. Stewart has them.
Mother: Really? Do you have them at school?
Child: uh uh.
A 3-second pause
Mother: Did you enjoy playing with your cards?

Figure 5.6d (Continued)

Dysfluent Discourse

Children are judged disorganized/disoriented in mildly stressful situations involving the parent (to date, either the Ainsworth Strange Situation, or the Clown Session devised by Main and Weston (1981)) when they show, with some intensity, any of a diverse array of specified behavior patterns indicative of conflict. These have been described by Main and Solomon (1986, 1990) and include: stilling and freezing of movement; stereotypies; simultaneous exhibition of contradictory tendencies (as, approaching with head averted); disordering of expected temporal sequences (crying and calling for the parent, then strongly avoiding the parent when the parent appears); direct indices of apprehension and confusion; and anomalous vocalizations.

Main and Hesse (1990) have suggested that many of these patterns seem to involve (a) the inhibition or contradiction of action as it is being undertaken, and (b) a possible experience of fear on the part of the infant. Thus, the disorganized infant is seen to rise to approach the parent on reunion, and then fall prone; to move toward the parent while averting the head; to move to lean head on the wall when apparently afraid of the stranger, but in the parent's presence; and frequently to freeze all movements, a behavior which to many ethologists seems indicative of fear, and an alternative to flight.

These disorganized/disoriented patterns of infant behavior have been found associated with the parent's history of attachment-related trauma, most usually involving unresolved mourning of attachment figures lost through death. There are indications, however, that the parent's (unresolved) experiences of sexual or physical abuse by their own parents may also be associated with the disorganized/disoriented behavior observed in their infants.

While interaction patterns between "D" infants and their parents have yet to be observed in the home situation, Main and Hesse (1990) have made informal observations suggesting that, in very subtle ways, the parents of "D" infants often behave in the Strange Situation as either frightening or frightened. "Frightening" behaviors on the parts of parents filmed in the Strange Situation are subtle, but include abrupt, unpredictable movement patterns; "looming"; rough movements of the infant's body; and peculiar intonations of voice. Indications of fearfulness on the part of the parent are generally subtle, but include seeking affection or attention from the infant in an unusual manner, and giving the infant the lead in the interaction while readily expressing a sense of having been rebuffed by the infant. Neither of these reactions to an infant is surprising, given the traumas which the parents have experienced themselves.

Given these descriptions of the children and their parents as observed in infancy, discourse descriptors are again consonant. We have not yet been able to provide sub-groups for the disorganized/disoriented infant category, so too there are only general descriptors for the dysfluent discourse category, without sub-groups. These are as follows:

1. Stumbling and false starts by both parent or child.
2. Topics largely focused upon relationship-relevant events, or upon evaluations of relationships.
3. Child frequently addresses the parent with imperatives.
4. The parent addresses the child with questions.
5. The parent is highly responsive to the child's conversational anomalies or unresponsiveness.
6. The parent responds passively to the child's steering of the conversation, that is, the parent does not elaborate or add with respect to a topic.
7. The parent indicates some disorientation; the child provides orientation.
8. The parent may offer unusually elaborate explanations when questioned by the child.

Figures 5.7a–5.7f give excerpts from several dysfluent transcripts.

Mother: Hi, Adam.
Child: Where's daddy?
Mother: He's, um, coming very soon. He went with, with, why, let's see, I was with Bonnie, and–
Examiner: Melinda
Mother: Melinda, yeah. And, um, he's talking with her, and he'll be back very soon. He's almost done.

Figure 5.7a D Discourse

Child: Mommy, watch this.
. . .
Mother: That's very nice. Did you play with sand?
Child: Yeah.
Mother: Oh. I thought that I would get to see the sandbox. Was it nice?
Child: Yeah.
Mother: But you like this better, huh?
Child: Yeah.
Mother: I see.
Child: Look at these guys. They can bend.
Mother: Yeah.
Mother: Can I see this one?
Child: Yeah.
Mother: Look at this one. Oh yeah. Right.
. . .
Mother: Ahh. Oh, you had cowboys, and–
Child: Yeah. I found some balls.
Mother: Some balls?
Child: Six.
Mother: Six of them?
Mother: Huh. In here?
Child: Yeah.
Mother: Oh, I see, were those in the sand?
Child: Yeah.
Mother: Yeah.
Child: Where's the king?
Mother: Which one was the king?

Figure 5.7a (Continued)

Child: Mom!
Mother: Hi.
Child: See, this is you, that's me, and Deirde, and um, a rainbow, and a house. You two in the house.
Mother: Who?
Child: That's, you and dad. Um, that's dad driving.
That's Vera, and Mom, that's you, and me, and Deirde.
. . .
Mother: Where's Lottie in this picture, Adam?
Child: Uh, Lottie? Oh, Lottie's not in that. You're all in the house.
Mother: Oh, Lottie's in the house?
Child: Yes, Lottie's in the house with you.

Figure 5.7b D Discourse

. . .
Child: Whee . . . Wanna play with me, mom, in the sandbox?
Mother: Sure. What are you doing?
Child: Playing with the animals. I'll get all the kings, all the castle things out.
Two-second pause
Child: Let's take all the castle guys out.
Mother: Oh, this is neat sand.
. . .
Child: Mom, ya wanna take all the animals out and set them up.
Mother: Okay, where, here?
. . .
Mother: Yeah. This is nice sand. This reminds me of the sand out at the ocean, out at the beach. Oh, I just love it.
Child: Okay. Let's take all the animals out and we can set them up.
Mother: Mmm, okay.
Child: In the sand.
Child: It's fun, isn't it?

Figure 5.7c D Discourse

Mother: Hey, that's neat, isn't it?
Child: Don't bother me, I'm making something.
Mother: You're making something. Okay.
Mother: That looks like fun. That looks like I'd like to jump in too and play.
Child: I'm making a sandcastle.
Mother: How do you like these little fellas, these little–
Child: Men.
Mother: Yeah, what are they called?

Figure 5.7d D Discourse

Mother: Hi. Oh, look at this. I didn't know there, did you know there was sand in the table where we were, where we were eating?
One-and-one-half-second pause
Mother: Oh.
Mother: Eve, what have you set up here? Hmm?
Three-and-one-half-second pause
Mother: What have you set up?
Mother: Here.
Six-second pause
Child: (mumbles)
Mother: I can't hear you.
Child: I made everything.

Figure 5.7e D Discourse

Mother: Oh, you made everything. You set out all of this?
Two-second pause
Mother: How neat.
Two-second pause
Mother: Can you tell me about it?
Three-and-one-half-second pause
Mother: Can you tell me about what you are doing?
Ten-and-one-half-second pause
Mother: Are you still setting up or are you almost finished?
Child: I'm still setting up.
Mother: Oh.
Two-second pause
Mother: Are you gonna tell me about this when you finish, then?
Twelve-second pause
Mother: Okay.

Figure 5.7e (Continued)

Mother: Oh boy, this is sure our king, queen, and castle day, isn't it?
Child: Mommy, do we have to go now?
Mother: In a little bit, when Dad's done. Why? Are you having fun?
Child: Because, you go over there. See, we're gonna make another–
Mother: Do you like it better when I'm not around?
Child: Yeah. Its easier for us to work.
Mother: Oh? Do I disrupt you?
Child: What?
Mother: Do I disrupt you?
Child: What?
Mother: I mean, do I make it so its harder for you to work?
Child: Yeah.
Mother: Oh, okay.
Child: (Mumbles).
Mother: Would you like for me to just be quiet and let you finish playing?

Figure 5.7f D Discourse

6 Instructions for the Classification of Children's Family Drawings in Terms of Representation of Attachment

Nancy Kaplan and Mary Main

This is a set of instructions for classifying the family drawings of children 5–7 years old in terms of their representation of attachment. The system was developed with the aim of capturing the quality of the child's attachment to their mother in infancy, assessed as secure, avoidant, ambivalent or disorganized/disoriented. In developing this system, we used our knowledge of individual differences in the organization of attachment relationships, as they appear in the Ainsworth Strange Situation categories and the Ainsworth home observations (Ainsworth et al., 1978) and in several new assessment procedures developed in our laboratory (the Adult Attachment Interview, the Separation Anxiety interview for 6-year olds, children's responses to a photograph of the family at 6 years, the child's response to reunion with the parent at 6 years and child–parent discourse during reunion, classification systems which are described briefly in Main et al. (1985)).

Earlier (Kaplan & Main, 1986), we reported success in a first classification attempt at (blind) identifications of drawings by 6-year-old children who had been secure, insecure-avoidant, and insecure-disorganized with mother as infants, obtaining a 76% hit-rate. However, until recently, we did not have a sufficient number of drawings by children who had been insecure-ambivalent in infancy to attempt to formalize instructions for their drawings.

We have recently completed our instructions for classifying children who were insecure-ambivalent/resistant with mother in infancy. We are now (1) engaged in studies of both short-term and long-term stability of children's drawing classifications; (2) attempting to predict sixth-year reunion attachment classifications from family drawings made in the school setting; (3) searching for differential errors in copy-drawings made by children in different attachment classifications; and (4) collecting and studying adult family drawings in conjunction with interviews concerning family and particularly family loss history.

Two attempts to replicate the association found in our sample between the child's Strange Situation classification to mother in infancy and the child's family drawing at 6 years of age are being undertaken in separate laboratories. While these studies are not complete, there are indications of strong predictability in a first study and little (insignificant) predictability in the second. In the first study, drawings were collected in the laboratory in the parent's

DOI: 10.4324/9781003569978-6

absence (as in our study), and strong stability of attachment organization from one to 6 years of age had also been established. In the second study, drawings were collected in the home, and the first-to-sixth-year stability of the child's attachment organization is unknown. For this reason, we urge researchers to collect the family drawings in the laboratory or school setting (and in the parent's absence) and to simultaneously assess sixth-year attachment organization to the mother wherever possible.

"Secure" drawings, drawing skill, and intelligence: Note on some possible confounds.

The drawings of 6-year-olds who were secure with mother in infancy (B), and particularly the drawings of 6-year-olds who were very secure with mother in infancy (B3) are recognized in large part for their realism, which includes not only representations of houses, and children's toys, but also completeness of human figure. Since completeness of human figure-drawing is a well-known measure of child intelligence (see Goodnow, 1977), we have cause to wonder whether symbolic processes or, instead, simply higher levels of intelligence underlie the association.

We have not attempted to assess intelligence for the Bay Area sample of children who provided the original drawings. In general, there is a weak, and usually insignificant, association between infant or child intelligence test scores and the "secure" vs. the "insecure" classifications. These differences are in the area of 5–7 points, which is no more than what could be accounted for by differences in levels of anxiety during testing. In the Bay Area sample, differences could be even less, since ours is a highly homogenous sample of families in which almost all parents had completed college, and many had graduate degrees and training.

Put somewhat differently, however, the question of the relationship between drawing skill and family representations is an intriguing one. We have begun to attempt to address it in a new sample of children, which we are studying first at 5 years of age. We have completed classifications of their family drawings. The traditional method of testing intelligence through child drawing involves a request to the child to Draw a Person (Goodnow, 1977), but, given the way in which representations of relationship appear in so many aspects of representation of persons, we doubted that the Draw a Person Test would do more than reflect again the child's attachment-influenced conceptualization of the person. Consequently, we requested the children in this new sample to draw a teddy bear set directly in front of them.

While analysis of this study is not complete, it is fair to say that (given our blind assessments of the "bear" drawings) there seems to be no relationship between the apparent skill, and completeness of drawing which appears in the drawing of the bear and in the family drawing. This is partly because several children whose family drawings were independently judged "secure" drew very poor, and obviously hasty, representations of the bear. More interesting is the fact that several children whose drawings were insecure – either disorganized, or incomplete as to body-part – drew relatively completely and skillful bear drawings. Thus, a child whose family had no arms drew arms and paws upon the bear. A child whose family was crossed-out and incomplete drew a complete and well-organized "bear" drawing.

Procedures

A laboratory or school setting in which the parents are absent (not in the same room as the child) should be used wherever possible. We used large sheets of art paper and a set of magic markers for our family drawings: however, a replication using 8½" × 11" paper and somewhat different watercolor pens has been successful. We recommend markers or pens which make bright, full lines, for example, lines resembling inks or watercolors.

The pens or markers should be set in front of the child in a set order on each occasion. It will be useful to the eventual study of color-use across samples if only the primary or close to primary colors are available to each child studied (6–8 markers). However, while in our previous studies, no flesh-tone was available, we are now planning to include this as a color.

The child should not be asked to attempt the family drawing until she seems at ease in the room and with the examiner. In the Berkeley study, a "warm-up" drawing was informally requested before the family drawing, for example, "would you like to draw something for me?" With respect to the family drawing, the examiner must make certain that several sheets of paper are visibly available to the child, so that the child who tends to want to re-start the family drawing on a second page can do so. It is important that the examiner is interested in the drawing, but takes the attitude that doing the drawing is a pleasant pastime and not any kind of an assignment, test, or task.

The researcher will want to know which figures in the drawing are which, what all the objects in the drawing represent, and ideally, which figure/object was drawn first and last. The examiner should maintain a friendly but non-interruptive interest in the drawing as the child draws it, so that asking who is who and what is what before the drawing is completed is usually inappropriate. When the drawing is completed, the examiner fills in, on the back of the drawing, an account of who is who in terms of family members, an explanation of any unexplained objects, and of the general setting of the drawing (e.g., "It's Halloween") when possible.

Video-taping in such a way that the creation of the child's in-process drawing, as well as the child's face and body, is in view is ideal. This takes two video cameras or a mirror reflecting the drawing. Audio-taping is helpful where video-taping is not possible.

Classification of Family Drawings

This classification system is based upon an assessment of the child's symbolic representation of attachment, rather than upon her skillfulness or technique.

In our most recent study, we are attempting to assess the child's skill at drawing apart from family drawings: while this study is still in progress, we have found several children whose family drawings appear much more primitive than their efforts to draw simple objects.

While we are providing as full a set of instructions as is possible at this time, we urge that coders, when making their judgments, draw upon their full understanding of individual differences in attachment. Not all children who were classified in a particular sub-group will produce a picture which conforms to our instructions; some drawings are particularly idiosyncratic or puzzling. The judge's broader understanding of attachment will be of use in these cases. Even in the less idiosyncratic pictures, using the specific instructions in combination with a full understanding of findings in attachment to date will contribute to an optimally informed judgment.

While we will ultimately use a new set of category headings for children's family drawings for the present time, we use the system of letters and numbers which refer to Strange Situation classifications and sub-classifications – the "A, B, C" system as presented in Ainsworth et al. (1978) and recently modified by Main and Solomon to include a "D" category (1986). *We* will refer to, for example, "B3" drawings to indicate commonalities discovered in the drawings of children who were classified as "very secure" (B3) with mother in infancy.

Note that our system does not include many simpler features, which would be expectable. For example, we find that the drawings of several children followed the "secure" pattern (in the following section) in overall quality, even though the children either included only themselves in the drawing or drew a family picture with the self absent. We found that these children had been secure with mother in infancy, as had one child who drew a drawing following the "secure" representational pattern which she described as being of a neighbor family.

The Family Drawings of Children Classified as "Secure" (B) With Mother in Infancy

Because sub-group B3 is the prototype of the B group, we begin with the instructions seeming best to describe the B3 drawings. These qualities are expected to pre-dominate in many of the sub-groups and to describe the qualities of many of the B drawings. However, the family drawings of children falling in different secure sub-groups in infancy can be distinguished at above a chance level, so sub-group instructions are given.

Characteristics of B3 Family Drawings and of the B Category in General

Overall impression. The observer's unstudied response to the drawing of the child who was classified as B3 in infancy includes the impression that the family (or the child) portrayed in the drawing is essentially happy. The drawing is realistic, calm, and human. In addition, many or most of the following descriptors fit to the drawing:

1. Figures are grounded or centered. They are firmly footed on some surface (imagined or drawn in), or, they are clearly secured near to page center.
2. There is a natural but not extreme proximity among family members. The picture gives the impression that the family members are accepting in a genuine way of one another, or even indirectly of an imagined observer. This is partly because of (a) a firm and (b) often open-armed, almost directly embracing stance taken by family members. There is (c) a natural proximity among family members, but (d) they are not placed so closely together that another could not join. Figures may lightly touch hands on occasion, but they are not all joined in one group and usually are not leaning together.
3. Often, not all family members are smiling: Sometimes, no family members are smiling. Where smiles do appear on some or all family members, they appear "genuine." Where family members are smiling, the smiles look genuine and do not have the quality exhibited in "happy-face" stickers.
4. Figures are individuated. Figures are not drawn identically. Facial expression and/or stance vary somewhat. The figures may be quite simple (heads attached directly to legs), but they are individuated if necessary by simple attributes (e.g., in a very simple drawing, a small infant figure might be shown as held by the mother).
5. Figures suggest movement. Figures are not rigid, restricted, or stiff.
6. "Real-world" elements are often present. Bicycles, a house, a lamp, the family dog, etc. may be present in the picture. These objects, however, do not pre-dominate over the picture. People if anything are predominant.
7. Figures are complete. More than for any other classification or subclassification, figures tend to be complete, with eyes, nose, mouth, hair, hands, and feet. To date, whole (major) parts of bodies (legs, arms) have not been drawn as missing on any figure in a B3 drawing, except when the child is clearly at an early stage of drawing in which legs are attached directly to heads.
8. The drawing may be highly imaginative or include fantasy elements. The child or family may be drawn in an unusual setting, for example, picking flowers or playing a game, or fantasy may be directly portrayed. However, for 6-year-olds, this is rare even in B3 drawings.
9. B3 family drawings, and B drawings in general, sometimes portray the child alone; portray child and mother with father missing; or even portray (deliberately) another family. No doubt, this has some significance, but appears that it does not mean that the child is insecure. What identifies the drawing as "B" despite the failure to include the child's whole family is the presence of the qualitative elements listed earlier.

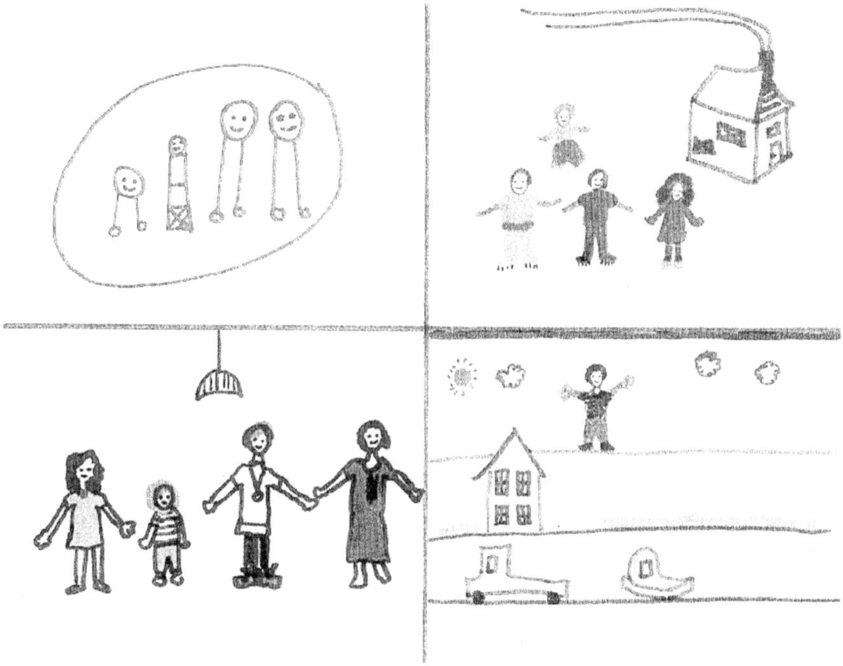

Figure 6.1 Examples of four drawings by 6-year-olds judged "B3" with mother in infancy

Figure 6.1 gives four examples of types of drawings shown by B3 6-year-olds. Note the way in which these drawings vary as well as the commonalities of composition as described earlier.

Sub-Group B1

These drawings have many elements described above as typifying group B drawings. However, as is well known, in terms of Strange Situation behavior, a B1 infant resembles an A infant in terms of failure to seek proximity and contact with the parent, but resembles a B3 infant in terms of making clear (through initiating distance interactions with the parent) its delight in the parent's return. In terms of the sixth-year drawing procedure:

1. The child presents himself or herself alone.
2. The drawing gives the impression that the child is ready for and/or would welcome interaction with others.
3. The drawing is solid, centered, and realistic and gives the impression of happiness. However, the child's arms are not placed in a fully embracing posture.

Sub-Group B2

Overall, the drawing qualifies for the general descriptors for "B" drawings given earlier. However, it also has some characteristics of the "A2" drawings to be described in the following section. This is particularly interesting because, within the Ainsworth Strange Situation, distinction between the A2 and B2 categories is well known to judges as being particularly difficult.

The overall impression presented to observers by the B2 drawing is that it is stolid, realistic, and firm and takes a positive stance. However, as compared to B3 drawings:

1. There is less individuation among family members.
2. There is a tendency for all family members to be smiling.
3. The figures are slightly stiff, and/or there is substantial distance between family members.
4. As we indicate, smiles and some stiffness of figure are shared with A2 drawings. However, there is greater individuation of figures, and smiling figures tend to show greater movement than in A2 drawings, or to be drawn in an embracing posture.

Sub-Group B4

The "B4" drawing has many elements of "B3" drawings. In the Ainsworth Strange Situation, however, the "B4" infant distinguishes itself from the B3 infant by a more whole-hearted focus upon the parent throughout the situation, and by a diminished interest (at least by the final reunion episode) in the return to play. Some disorganization in behavior is also occasionally observed in these infants, but it differs from that of true "D" infants in that it is either very slight, or is quickly succeeded by an effort to regain proximity to the parent.

As we might expect, given the Strange Situation behavior of these children as infants, there is also some resemblance in B4 drawings to drawings by children falling in the C and/or D categories, as well as to children judged B3:

1. Figures may be more expressive and idiosyncratic than is expected in a B3 drawing.
2. Bodies may be round, and facial features may be emphasized. However, in contrast to the C drawings, there is nothing unpleasant in this emphasis.
3. Differences of size among family members may be pleasantly exaggerated, with some figures large and some small. In contrast to the C drawings, however, there is something humorous or simply expressive in these size differences.
4. As in some "D" drawings, there may be an impression of chaos or disorganization, but this is overridden by the human and perhaps personal qualities of the drawing, for example, the person or persons presented.

5. As in the "over-bright" "D" drawings, there may be brightly colored, gay elements – for example, balloons or flowers – but while these have an element of slightly excessive cheer, they do not override the essential realism of the drawing.
6. In some B4 drawings, and to date not in others, a figure may be shown with an anxious or pained smile, for example, a smiling face with worry-lines around the eyes. These faces suggest to the observer that the stress that the child experiences is humanly contained and expressed. Thus, rather than adding ominous disorganized elements to the drawing – as does the child who was disorganized/disoriented as an infant – the "B4" child in this drawing indicates the experience of stress directly, and without translating it into symbolic form. Following are examples of two "worried" faces drawn by B4 children (Figure 6.2).

Figure 6.3 illustrates several of the types of B drawings observed in our own and other samples. In the upper left-hand corner is a B1 drawing; on the right, a B2 drawing; and left and right of page bottom illustrate two B4 drawings.

The Family Drawings of Children Classified as "Insecure-Avoidant" (Group A) With Mother in Infancy

Overall, these drawings appear as an attempt to present a positive picture of an invulnerable and "happy" individual or family. The emphasis on happiness or invulnerability in these drawings is to be expected based upon (a) the Strange Situation behavior of the insecure-avoidant infant,

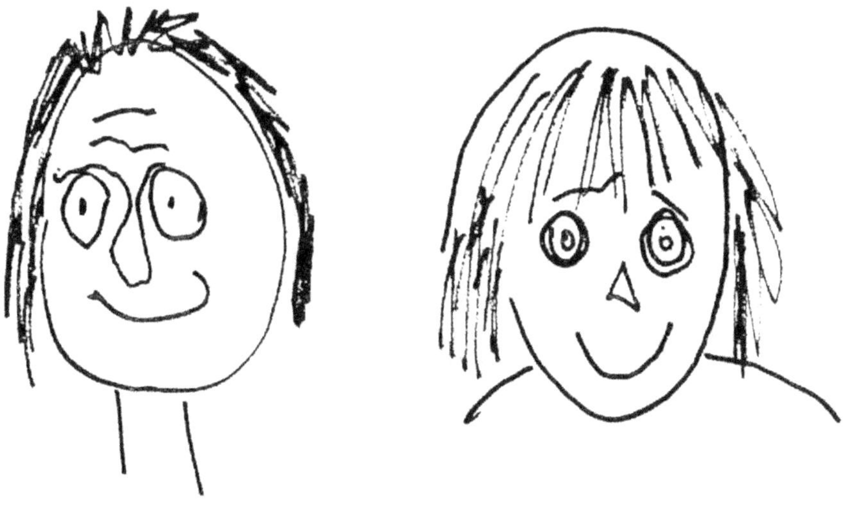

Figure 6.2 "Worried" faces drawn by B4 children

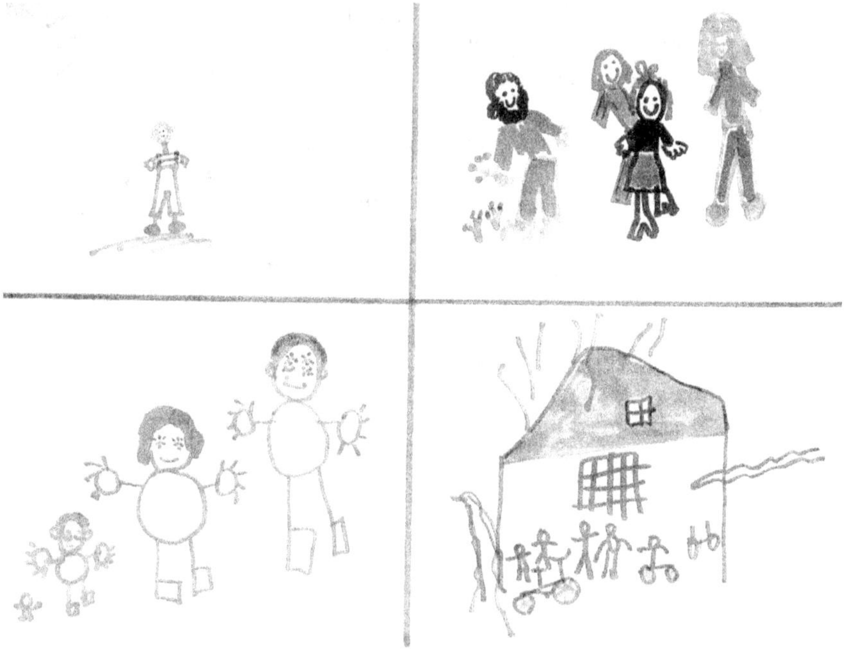

Figure 6.3 Examples of drawings by 6-year-olds judged B1, B2, and B4 with mother in infancy. Upper left corner = B1; upper right corner = B2. Both drawings on the lower half of the page are by children judged B4 with mother in infancy

in which distress is not shown, (b) the observations of Klaus Grossmann and his colleagues in Regensburg, South Germany, in which close analysis of both the Strange Situation and of free play indicated that mothers responded to insecure-avoidant infants when they indicated happiness, but not when they indicated distress, and (c) the characteristics of the parents of insecure-avoidant infants discovered within adult attachment analysis, in which the adult frequently describes the self as strong and the parents as unusually excellent. The Group A drawings are characterized by many or all of the following features:

1. Arms are either:
   a. absent on one or all family members, or
   b. are portrayed in postures not suitable for holding.

   Note: Very rarely, a 6-year-old is still in the "tadpole" stage of drawing, in which heads are attached to legs, and arms are therefore absent. The judge should be able to determine, however, from the overall quality of the drawing, whether the child had the capacity to draw arms or not. As an obvious example, where legs and feet are well drawn; or where some figures have arms; or where drawing ability seems high in general, the absence of arms in a particular drawing is significant.

2. Lack of individuation of family members. The observer may have the impression that figures were drawn automatically, one after the other, without attention to individual characteristics.
3. Figures do not appear to be affected by one another or to be related to one another.
4. Smiles, often apparently somewhat automatically drawn, are often present on every family member.
5. Figures are portrayed as stiff and without movement.

Sub-Group A1

In the Ainsworth Strange Situation, the A1 infants are extremely avoidant. Typically, they not only do not cry when mother leaves them alone with the stranger, but they also do not cry when left completely alone. On reunion, they show not even the subtle signs of proximity-seeking or anger shown by the A2 infants.

The A1 drawings share the general characteristics of "A" drawings described earlier. In addition:

1. The picture gives the impression of isolation, loneliness, or absence of connectedness – despite its overall "up" or "positive" stance. Sometimes, this is shown by great distance between family members; sometimes, by the child being portrayed alone; sometimes, by the fact that, although a "ground" and a "sky" are present, the family seems to float in the air.
2. On close examination, there is something about the drawing that is not solid, and that does not convey an impression of having been drawn with ease or calm. The marks made on the paper may be tense; the figures themselves may appear extremely stiff and tense; and some faint ominousness may be present as well.

Figure 6.4 gives examples of drawings by several 6-year-olds who were classified as "A1" with parents in infancy. Note the impression of isolation.

Sub-Group A2

The A2 drawings share the general characteristics of group A drawings, described earlier. However, our Berkeley follow-up study has showed (Main et al., 1985) that children who were A2 as infants were functioning adequately on diverse assessments at six. In addition, their parents, though ultimately classified through the adult attachment analysis as "dismissing of attachment", expressed in interview much more of the sense of the influence of attachment-related experiences upon development, and more feeling, than

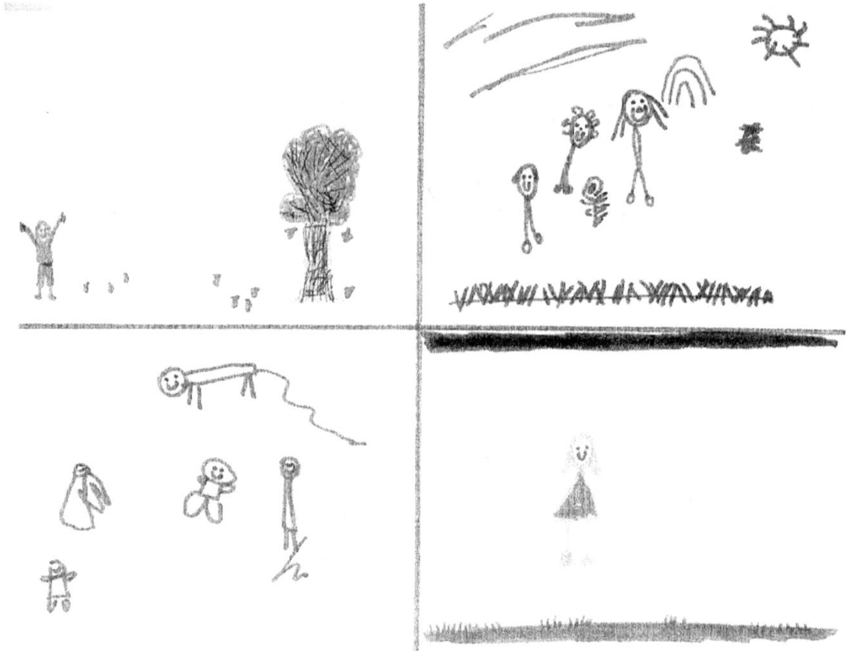

Figure 6.4 Four examples of drawings by 6-year-olds classified A1 with mother in infancy

the parents of infants classified as "A1" in infancy. The drawings of their infants as 6-year-olds show the following characteristics:

1. The drawing is more realistic than an A1 drawing, and usually does not contain even subtly ominous elements. The drawing is likely to be centered and grounded.
3. However, unlike a "B" drawing, events and movement are absent. The observer has the impression that the picture, though positive and sometimes solid, is empty. The impression ultimately given is that there is nothing happening.

Figure 6.5 illustrates several examples of A2 drawings by 6-year-olds. The reader attempting to learn the system should compare the qualities of these drawings with both the B2 and the A1 drawings.

The Family Drawings of Children Classified as "Insecure-Ambivalent/Resistant" (C) With Mother in Infancy

These family drawings are the most heterogeneous and difficult to characterize. They share many features with "B" and with "A" drawings. For

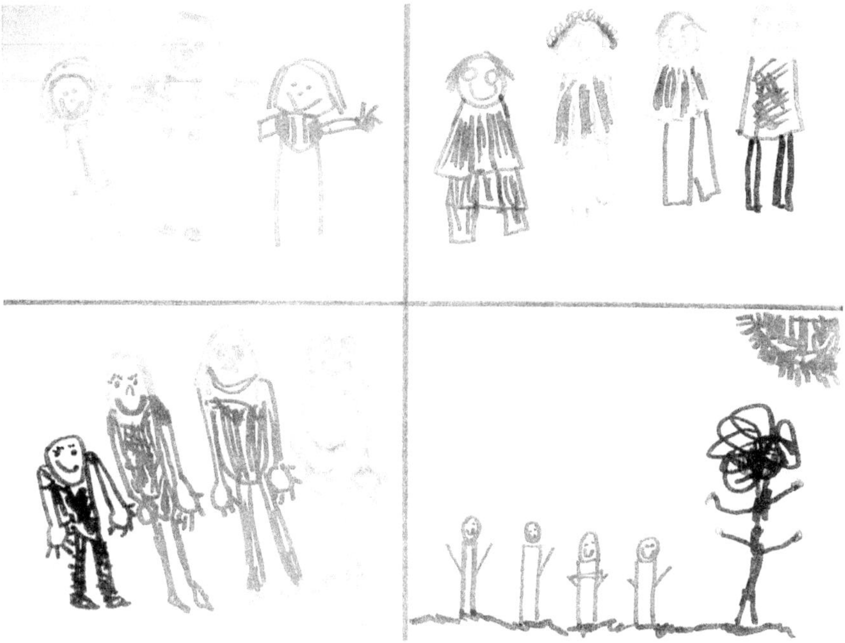

Figure 6.5 Four examples of drawings by children classified A2 with mother in infancy

example, many drawings by children classified C with mother in infancy present the child's arms in an embracing posture, and many or all figures are often presented smiling. On the whole, however, family drawings made by children who were classified C with mother in infancy tend to emphasize upon size of figures (very large or very small); emphasize upon proximity to and/or the inaccessibility of individuals (clinging and melding together or separated by a barrier); and emphasis and exaggeration of particular vulnerable soft body parts and facial features (the belly and lower body, eyes, and nostrils).

Informally interpreted, there seems in these drawings to be an *emphasis upon vulnerability*. This impression is based upon consideration of vulnerability as shown in:

huge parental or family figures – figures which almost fill the page and seem overwhelming

or extremely tiny family figures – figures which appear overwhelmed by the spaces surrounding them

figures placed in the corners of the page, or top or bottom, again appearing overwhelmed by the surround

exaggerated emphasis upon "soft" features of the body, as, large round stomachs and exposed belly buttons.

In some drawings, all of these characteristics may be combined, for example, some figures huge and some tiny; two figures clinging together and another seen at the opposite side of the page; and large bellies and large eyes.

As in the Strange Situation, there is little difficulty in distinguishing between A and C, but distinctions between B and C can be difficult. In addition, distinctions between the drawings of children who were classified in sub-group C1 vs. sub-group C2 in infancy have not been possible to date. In general, we can specify the following features, only a few of which may be present in any particular drawing:

1. Unusually large or unusually small figures, or (rarely) both in a single drawing. As though in further emphasis, figures may be placed off-center, as, in the far lower left-hand corner.
2. Family figures placed extremely close together, bodies overlapping, or leaning together, clinging, or universally holding hands.
3. Figures are portrayed as separated by a barrier, as, figures shown on either side of a large house.
4. Emphasis upon the *belly, and/or lower body,* shown in one of the following features:

    a. large, round bellies
    b. belly buttons drawn in
    c. figures which become big from the waist down, moving from a small upper body through large lower body and still larger legs and feet, as though the body is being drawn from below.

    Note: The latter feature also occurs in some B3 and B4 drawings.

Special Features

The following special features appear in some drawings by children in the C classification. *Item a* appears frequently and distinctively enough to be considered a serious candidate for pathognomic category marker. We mention *items b* because as more drawings are collected, these features may appear more often in C than other drawings: However, they are rare in our present collection of C drawings, and do appear in children in other categories (especially, in B4 drawings).

a. An unusual, striking, and sometimes ominous slant to the neck/head relative to the shoulders and rest of the body, as in Thai dance or other dance movements imitating the tracking-mesmerizing movement. To date, this has appeared in just under half of drawings by children who were classified as C in infancy, and in no others. Sometimes the head angle appears less ominous than simply peculiarly slanted or sharply cocked. Figure 6.6 contains several drawings which illustrate this peculiar slant of the neck.

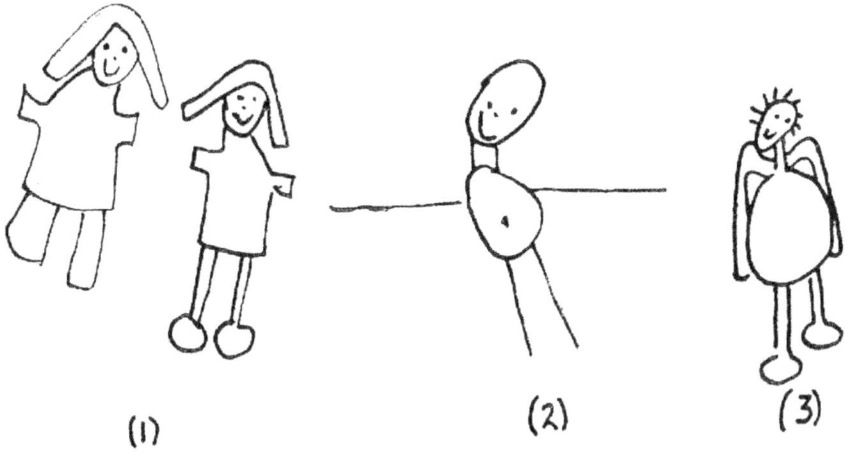

Figure 6.6 Children's drawings illustrating slant of the neck

b. Exaggeration of the personal features of the face – as seen in some B4 drawings – but, in contrast to B4 drawings, the effect is unpleasant. For example, a figure may be drawn with large eyes and eyelashes and with circle-noses with prominent round nostrils. Below is a drawing (Figure 6.7), which illustrates this unusual facial configuration.

Figure 6.8 presents examples of the drawings of several children who were categorized as falling within Group C. Note again the unusual heterogeneity of drawing type (comparable to that shown in group B4).

The Family Drawings of Children Judged Disorganized/Disoriented With Mother in Infancy

The family drawings of children who were disorganized/disoriented with mother in infancy *cannot be distinguished from others in the same terms in which we distinguish A, B, and C drawings*: Indeed, any of the qualities which we have described as characterizing A, B, and C drawings may be found in the drawings of children who were categorized as D as infants. This makes sense, in that any of the major attachment categories may become disorganized (Main & Solomon, 1986, 1990).

Most of the drawings of these children are distinguished from others either by (a) simple disorganization of elements, as scratching-out and re-starts, or (b) by adding unexpected elements to the drawing or omitting expected elements, as standing family members on a row of hearts, or putting only one eye in a head. (Very rarely, the family drawing of a child who was classified D with mother in infancy can be distinguished from others simply because it fails to fit any (A, B, C, or D) of the described patterns).

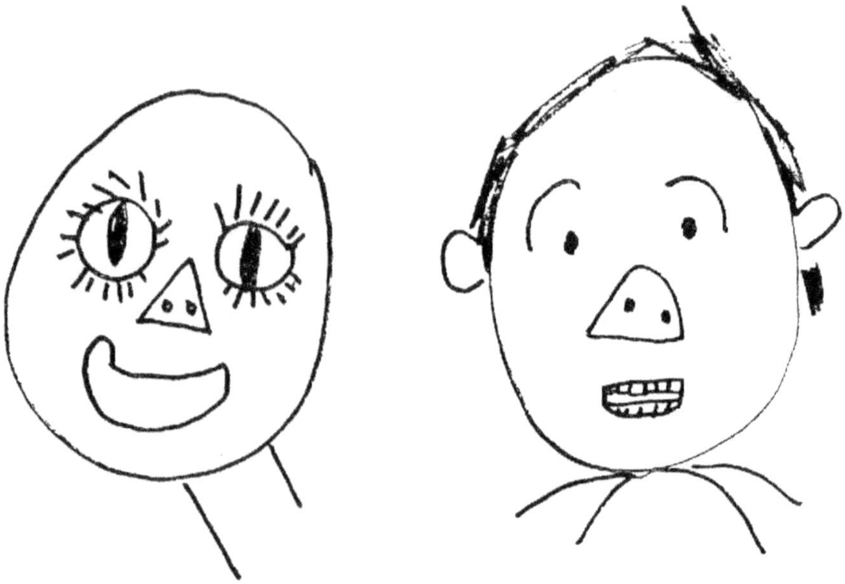

Figure 6.7 Children's drawings illustrating the exaggeration of the personal features of the face

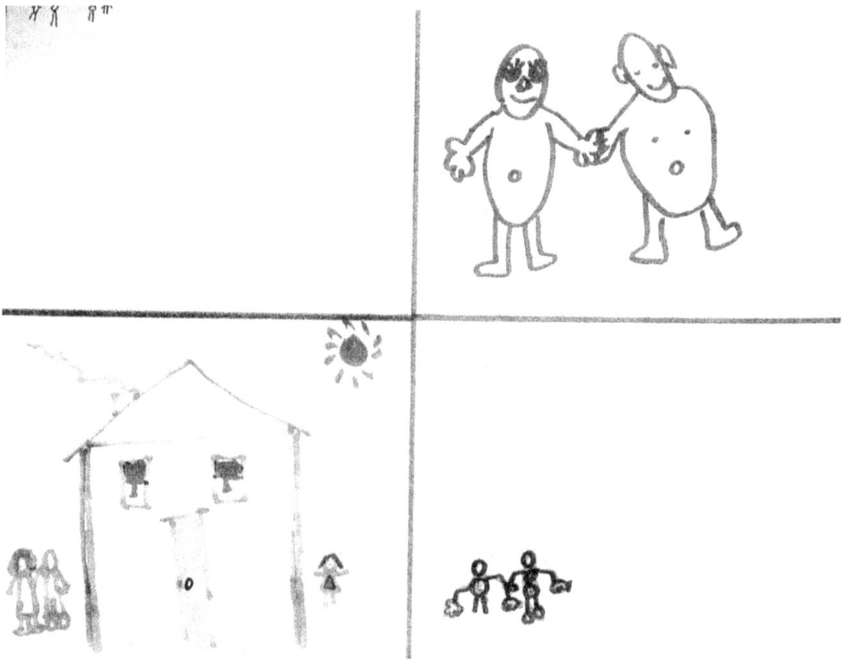

Figure 6.8 Examples of drawings from several children who were categorized as falling within Group C

The family drawings of children who were disorganized/disoriented with mother in infancy can be described as falling into one of the following three patterns (patterns 1 and 2 may be combined in a single picture).

I. *Ominous, irrational, or disorganized.* The family picture is ominous, foreboding, and/or directly disorganized.

1. Strange inexplicable marks may be added to the picture, as, a crossed-out heart in the sky, a skeleton, or a figure with wolf-like teeth.
2. Unfinished objects or figures may be present, as, a small head on the ground, an ear, etc.
3. The child may scratch out a figure in the picture or part of the picture and re-start it on the same page or on a separate page, essentially in part destroying or rejecting part of the work. To date this has occurred only in children who were disorganized/disoriented with mother in infancy.

Note: Children who were classified A1 or C2 with mother in infancy may also include strange features or inexplicable marks in their drawings but (a) nothing is actually scratched out and (b) the features are more unlikely than they are frightening or ominous.

II. *Over-bright family pictures.* Excessive or almost irrational sweetness is added to the picture or is placed near a person in the picture. Thus, the family may be pictured as standing on a row of hearts; a huge sun with a smiling face may dominate the picture; hearts and flowers may be literally displayed; a sun may be placed very close to a human head. At first glance, the picture may simply appear very sweet or very cheerful, but on closer examination, it contains irrational or unrealistic elements, that is, people do not stand on hearts or have suns directly next to their heads.

III. *Unclassifiable.* The picture is not disorganized, ominous, or overly bright. However, it also does not fit with the descriptions given of A, B, and C drawings, but may have characteristics of all three types of drawings.

Figure 6.9 gives examples of the three types of "D" drawings. In the upper left-hand corner is a drawing considered over-bright; to the upper right and lower left are drawings considered ominous; and the drawing on the lower right does not fit either to the A, B, C, or D classifications, but has some elements of all. The drawing was judged blind: The child was later discovered to indeed have been disorganized/disoriented during infancy.

Note: When giving the family drawing any kind of a "D" classification (ominous, over-bright, or unclassifiable) give in addition the "A," "B," or "C" classification which seems best to fit. Thus, the row of identical, well-centered, stiff, smiling figures standing on a row of hearts with a bright sun over one head would be classified D (over-bright)/A2.

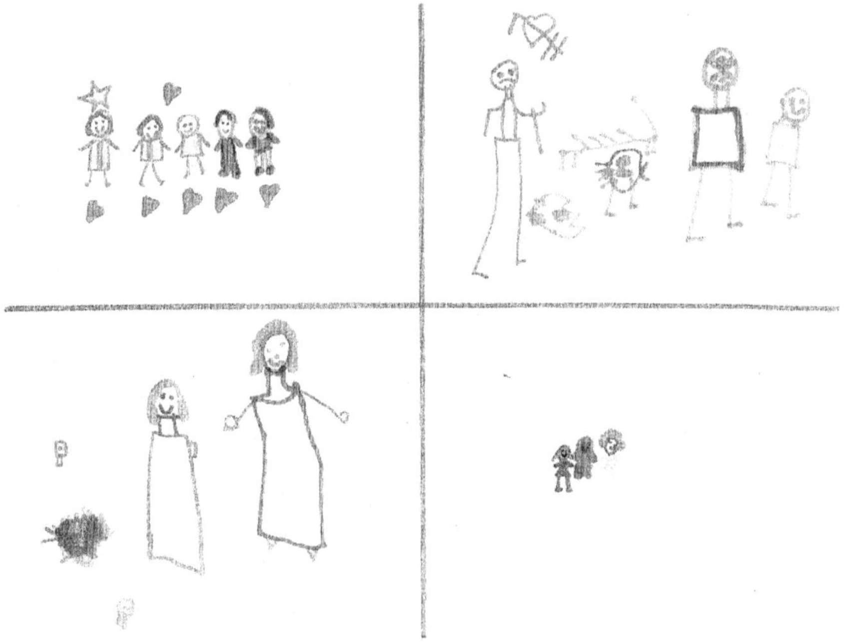

Figure 6.9 Four examples of drawings by 6-year-olds judged disorganized/disoriented (D) with mother in infancy. An "over-bright" drawing is in the upper left-hand corner; "ominous" drawings are in the upper right-hand corner and lower left-hand corner of the page. An "unclassifiable" drawing is in the lower right-hand corner

7 Assessments of Child–Parent Attachment at Six Years of Age

Mary Main and Jude Cassidy

These systems are designed to assess individual differences in children's (video-taped) responses to reunion with the parent following a separation of approximately 1 hour. We have developed three measures to assess the child's response. The first is a 9-point scale assessing overall apparent *security or confidence* in the relationship. The second is a 7-point scale assessing the degree to which the child appears to *avoid* physical proximity to or emotional interaction and confrontation with the parent.

The third assessment is a *classification* system intended to identify the apparent organization of the attachment relationship during this reunion episode: *secure, insecure-avoidant, insecure-ambivalent, insecure-controlling,* and *insecure-unclassified.*

The *secure, insecure-avoidant,* and *insecure-ambivalent* sixth-year categories are equivalent to the A, B, C categories developed by Ainsworth for infant Strange Situation behavior (Ainsworth et al., 1971). Recently, Main and Solomon (1986) have identified a "D" category of infant Strange Situation behavior, currently conceived as a disorganization of underlying A, B, or C categories. Disorganized ("D") 1-year-olds are assigned at once to the D "category" and simultaneously to a best-fitting A, B, or C Strange Situation category. Thus, judges examining Strange Situation behavior of a particular infant may first determine that the infant's behavior is disorganized: At the same time, however, they assign or "force" the infant to an A, B, or C category.

Similarly, a 6-year-old who fails to fit readily to the A, B, or C sixth-year equivalents will have been described by the system as either insecure-controlling/directing or insecure-unclassified. This 6-year-old is simultaneously assigned to a best-fitting secure, insecure-avoidant, or insecure-ambivalent category.

Our classification system includes sub-categories as well as major categories. Some of these sub-categories have direct first-year equivalents, as, the sixth-year sub-category, neutral-avoidant.

Inter-judge reliability. Inter-judge reliability was established for the Charlottesville tapes by two judges, who independently (without conferencing) classified and rated each 6-year-old (N = 50). Inter-rater reliability for security was $r = 0.80$; for avoidance, it was $r = 0.92$; and for the classifications, it was

DOI: 10.4324/9781003569978-7

76% agreement using four classes and 84% using the "forced" A, B, C classification system.

Issues of Predictability

In earlier and current reports, we have compared assessments of infant Strange Situation behavior to mother and (independently) to father at 1 year of age to reunion behavior toward the same parent at 6 years of age. Our report concerned a sample of 34 upper-middle class, Bay Area families who had remained intact (parents neither separated nor divorced) over the 5-year period between our infancy and our sixth-year studies. Independent judges working without knowledge of one another's assessments discovered substantial (r = 0.77) correlations between security shown on reunion with the mother at 1 year of age (assessed as very secure, secure, or insecure) and security at 6 years of age, and between avoidance of mother on reunion at 1 year and again at 6 years of age (r = 0.63). The hit-rate for 12 month to sixth-year major attachment classification in this upper middle-class sample was over 80% with mother, with children who were secure with mother in infancy being judged secure at 6 years of age, children who were insecure-avoidant being judged avoidant, and children who were insecure-disorganized in infancy being found insecure-directing or insecure-unclassified at 6 years of age. Corresponding relationships between 12-month and sixth-year reunion behavior to the father were weak (p.05) or insignificant (e.g., avoidance of the father at 6 years could not be predicted from avoidance of father during the infancy period).

Recently, Jude Cassidy has assessed stability in conjunction with her doctoral thesis conducted at the University of Virginia. Fifty 6-year-olds in her Charlottesvile sample were seen with mother two times (1 month apart) in a study, which compared sixth-year child–mother attachment classifications to the child's self-concept. The two reunions were assessed by independent judges. Ratings for security and avoidance were stable over the 1-month period (r (50) = 0.62 for security, 0.66 for avoidance). Using the four major sixth-year classifications (secure, avoidant, ambivalent, controlling), Cassidy found 62% (31 out of 50) of her subjects stable in terms of a four-category system classification across the 1-month period. However, the insecure-directing and insecure-unclassified categories were unstable over the 1-month period. This instability in the insecure-directing category – the equivalent to infancy category "D" – may have been due to differential stress in the laboratory procedure at the two periods (refer to the section "Procedures").

Each subject in the Cassidy sample who was judged insecure-directing or insecure-unclassified was simultaneously assigned to a "forced" or "best-fitting" A (avoidant), B (secure), or C (ambivalent) category. We estimated stability a second time, with every child in the sample "forced" into one of the three central categories at each time period. Stability using an "A, B, C" classification system was 84% (42 of the 50 children in the sample remained in the same one of three categories). Using this forced-choice system, 38 out of the 50 (76%) children were placed in the same one of eight traditional sub-categories (A1, A2, B1, B2, B3, B4, C1, C2) in both sessions.

The two studies cited above demonstrate an impressive predictability in attachment organization with respect to the mother in two white, middle-class samples. However, they are concerned exclusively with white, middle-class populations and include one sample (the Bay Area sample) deliberately selected for the absence of events known to have a deleterious effect upon attachment organization. Sample I informed us regarding the patterns of reunion behavior to mother which developed between 1 and 6 years of age in children from stable families, when attachment organization was largely undisturbed by major events external to mother–child interaction. Our system was developed using this stable population.

Applying the system developed using Sample I to Sample II, we were able to establish good reliability, and found surprising "A, B, C" stability using the forced-choice system. This sample also suggested surprising viability for the "A, B, C" sub-group system, since judges were reliable with respect to sub-group placement, and impressive stability in sub-group placement was demonstrated across the 1-month period.

Both Study I and Study II raise important questions for researchers in attachment. First, we should ask whether there is really a difference in predictability of reunion responses over the 5-year period for father–child as opposed to mother–child dyads. Second, we will need to examine the meaning of the instability in the insecure-directing category found in Sample II. We have at present a number of hypotheses, which can be ruled out only by further study. One is that "directing" behavior is very sensitive to procedures; another, that we had simply failed to recognize the logical necessity of devising a set of "directing-like" sub-categories, for example, A(d), B(d), and C(d) for each of the A, B, and C categories. A substantial number of the "unstable" controlling-directing children in the Cassidy sample showed some controlling/directing behavior in both sessions.

Transformation in relationships over a 5-year period: Addressing issues of homotypic vs. heterotypic continuity. In the Berkeley sample, we found different kinds of changes in sixth-year reunion behavior depending upon the child's original Strange-Situation classification. As expected, very few 6-year-olds showed distress during separation from the parent, few touched the parent on reunion, and very few maintained contact with the parent. Instead, children who had been *secure* with the mother in infancy actively initiated interaction with the mother, or were highly responsive to the parent's initiations. Children who had been *avoidant* of the mother in infancy actively minimized interaction with the parent at six, and some subtly moved away from the parent on reunion. At six, however, children who had been avoidant as 1-year-olds spoke (minimally) when seriously pressed to do so by the parent. Failure to respond occurred only in circumstances in which the child could look busy or in which the child could reasonably have failed to hear the parent. It seems likely that by six, the child has learned that not-speaking when pressed to speak is confrontational rather than minimizing of relationship.

Children who had been categorized as *ambivalent* and children who had been categorized as *disorganized* in infancy showed unexpected behavior changes between 1 and 6 years of age. Six-year-olds who had been *ambivalent* in infancy showed the hostility and/or passivity characterizing the insecure-ambivalent infant, but *in addition, they showed moderate avoidance.* Similar findings have been reported by attachment researchers working in Minnesota (Vaughn et al., 1979). These workers reported that several infants classified as ambivalent at 12 months were classified as avoidant 6 months later. Thus, in two separate studies conducted over differing time periods, moderate to substantial avoidance has appeared in children categorized as ambivalent at 12 months of age.

The most striking transformation occurred in children who had been determined to be *disorganized/disoriented* with mother or father in infancy. The great majority of these children were directing and/controlling toward the parent 5 years later, that is, exceptionally organizing with respect to the parent and the parent's activities. We interpret this change in light of the association between infant disorganization and parental experience of trauma (e.g., early loss of a parent) which we have reported elsewhere. The parent's disorganization, fearfulness, and perhaps occasional frightening behavior is reflected in disorganization and disorientation when the offspring is an infant. Later, however, the child seems to enter into a kind of solution to the problem presented by the parent who is disorganized or disoriented by trauma – taking care of, directing, and organizing the parent through role-reversal.

Procedures Used in the Assessment of Sixth-Year Attachment

The directions and principles for this reunion procedure vary in important ways from those involved in the most well-known separation-and-reunion procedure, namely, the Ainsworth Strange Situation. We have reason to think that conduct of the sixth-year procedure affects the child's behavior strongly, such that variations from the procedure suggested here may affect the ability of this classification system to accurately reflect important qualities of the parent–child relationship. We summarize our directions as follows:

1. *The reunion should take place in a room, which provides ample room for child and parent to move about while remaining on camera.* The furniture should be arranged so that both child and parent have a choice of places to position themselves, and so that entertaining objects are available in several places. A larger room than the usual "Strange Situation" laboratory room is therefore needed.

   Rationale. Both child and parent need options regarding where they are to sit or stand during the reunion. This lowers both self-consciousness and camera consciousness. An avoidant child needs to be able to move away from the parent. If uncomfortable in a given position, both individuals need to be able to shift.

2. *The child should have numerous highly attractive toys and other objects available.* In the Berkeley studies, we had a castle with dragons, knights, king, queen, and horses against the wall, and a sandbox with numerous fantasy-play objects available. In Regensburg, South Germany, the child had available large, attractive construction toys, a tea set, and a group of hand puppets arranged on a bookcase, which could serve as a puppet theater.

   Rationale. Parent and child need "topics" for discussion on reunion, and this naturally includes the toys in the room and what the child has been doing with them. Well-selected toys provide parent and child with the opportunity for playing together during the reunion, for example, using the sandbox together, or playing puppet theater together. Finally, and perhaps most importantly, a child who wishes to avoid the parent needs a selection of objects to attend to. When all such objects are absent, the child cannot avoid the parent.

3. *The child should have been engaged in free play with these toys, in the company of an entirely pleasant and responsive examiner, for at least 20 minutes prior to the moment of reunion.* It is very important to accuracy of classification that the child be relaxed, occupied, and as happy as possible when the parent makes her or his entrance. As soon as the free play period begins, the examiner should make it clear to the child that, whatever tasks have preceded these final minutes, her sole concern now and for the remainder of the period is that the child enjoys herself. The child should understand that all tasks and tests are behind her: She can play as she likes until the parent returns, with the examiner participating now and then if the child wishes.

   We do not attempt in any way to "stress" 6-year-olds regarding the whereabouts or the return of the parent in the sixth-year procedure. These children should under no conditions worry about the return of the parent, and tests and tasks used by the researcher even prior to the free play session should not be stressful.

   Rationale. In the Strange Situation, stress is used to heighten individual differences in attachment organization. In this procedure, in contrast, we make the child as comfortable as possible during separation. If the child is very pleasantly occupied, we may find either that the parent's return is not disappointing (secure children), or that the child finds it somewhat troubling (insecure children). The reunion is maximally informative under these conditions.

   The endeavor is to see what the "image" of the parent calls up for a child who is in a relaxed and relatively happy state of engagement in play. Many children who have been left in unpleasant or tiring circumstances will show some punitive, semi-controlling behavior on reunion with the parent. We are attempting to structure the situation so that the child has no immediate cause for being in a poor mood, depressed, or negative toward the parent.

4. *Parental reunion behavior is not controlled and the reunion is not emphasized to the parent in any way.* The parent's return to the playroom is casual. Although the parent will have been informed long previously that everything taking place in the playroom is being filmed, the return to the playroom is not emphasized. The parent, with all her own tasks behind her, simply joins the child and child examiner in the playroom while the adult examiner gathers together the video consent forms. The atmosphere is not that this is the vital moment of reunion, but that the sessions are over.

   Rationale. Any effort to direct the reunion behavior of the parent with children of this age is almost certain to result in socially strange behavior on the part of the parent. Our effort here is to have the child in as stress-free a setting as possible at the time of reunion with the parent. Following the classification system, we need to be certain that the child is not, for example, avoiding the parent or being punitive toward the parent because the parent is behaving strangely. Only a completely natural and unstructured reunion situation assures this outcome.

5. *The child examiner remains in the room during the reunion, to increase the naturalness of the situation and to ease self-consciousness on the part of the parent.* Since the parent has been engaged in other tasks or interviews until this moment – and is now about to leave the laboratory – it is natural to simply thank the parent for participation and inform her that she can return to the playroom and get ready to leave with the child. Beyond her natural greeting to the parent, the child examiner should then be simply quietly responsive rather than directive. She is friendly and polite, but not really open to conversation with the parent in that she is quietly occupied with a barely noticeable, non-interruptive task of her own. If the parent elects to address the examiner rather than the child, the examiner should interact naturally. Otherwise, she should simply busy herself with some kind of interruptible task of her own, such as quietly sorting through the toys in the sandbox. The examiner should not move about much. Again, she should appear occupied enough that the parent feels no social necessity to interact with her.

   She acts, correctly, as though she is not an important person at the moment, and although she responds if the parent speaks, she does not ask questions herself nor extend any conversation between herself and the parent or between herself and the child. Her look of friendly but absent unimportance should be sufficient to prevent the parent from addressing the first usual question "what have you been doing in here?" to anyone but the child. Such initial questions of parent to child or to the room's occupants should never be addressed by the examiner. At the same time, the mildly occupied examiner should not make these last few minutes seem like an experiment. If the parent addresses her, she should be friendly.

In our Berkeley study, 6-year-old children had visited the laboratory together with both parents. Our reunions were designed to allow one parent to enter first, followed by the second parent several minutes later (mother was the first to enter the room for half our families). After the second parent had been in the room for approximately 3 minutes, the experimenter re-entered the room to ask the parents to sign additional release forms for the video-taping.

When the second parent returned to the room in the Berkeley study, the room contained the playmate, the child, and the first parent. There is a good bit of greeting to be done in such a situation, but our impression is that this kind of overloaded cast of characters helps to keep the situation natural. In the Berkeley study, mothers and fathers were first to enter the room in alternating sessions, so that mothers were first (fathers were first) for half the sample. The first-year to sixth-year classification hit-rate was virtually identical for parents entering the room first or second at 6 years of age.

Video-Taping. Split-screen video-taping is ideal for this situation, with one camera focused upon the door for parent's entrance while one camera is focused upon the child. We suggest, however, that the camera focused upon the door (parent) not be moved to follow the parent, unless the laboratory has use of a one-way vision mirror. This camera movement is immediately noted by the parent, and will surprise her as well as making her self-conscious at the moment of greeting. The only mobile camera should be the one which is obviously focused upon and following the child.

The examiner should be instructed to have the child positioned so that her reaction to the parent's entrance can be recorded. This should not be especially difficult, since playroom activities have most likely been video-taped throughout the separation period, with emphasis upon filming of the child. However, the examiner should be aware of the approximate time of the parent's expected entrance and should be alert to sounds of the returning parent and examiner. The child should not have her back to the camera at this time, so, the examiner may need to re-position her. If she hears the parent in the hall, the examiner should, draw the child's attention to the parent's return ("Oh, it's your mother") so that the camera can capture the child's response. The examiner should not, however, obscure the moment of greeting: If the examiner does not notice the parent's return until the parent is just outside the door, she should leave it to the child to note the return herself.

For laboratories using only one camera, focus should be kept fairly continually upon the child. Use as wide-angle a lens as possible, however, so that some interaction can be captured. The camera should be continually upon the child, especially for the first minute. The shot should be a close-up. After that point, if the parent is close to the child, the camera can pull back to include both. If the parent is far away, the camera can quickly pan to her for a few seconds every 20–30 seconds.

Preparation for Coding

Making a *verbatim transcript* of the speech of all participants, together with brief notes as needed regarding non-verbal behavior, is of invaluable assistance in further coding. *Coding* of the child's response to reunion should begin approximately 15 seconds before the door opens in order to assess the child's reaction when she learns that the parent is entering the room. In studies involving two entrances, coding continues until the second parent is entering or is about to enter the room. Any further interaction with the first parent is no longer taken into consideration. Coding with respect to the second parent begins, as soon as the child realizes that the parent is about to enter the room and continues through the dyad's exit. *Exit behavior is of real interest.* Some parents have difficulty persuading the child to leave the room: Individual differences in negotiation around leave-taking can reveal important aspects of the relationship.

All reunion episodes for a given sample should be spliced together. The splicing begins 30 seconds before the parent's entrance so that the coder can have a sense of the child's mood and activities before the 15 or so seconds in which she is aware of the coming return of the parent.

As work on individual cases begins, the judge should first assign the rating for avoidance; then the rating for security; and finally assign the classification. We have found rating and classifying a given case takes from 1 to 2 hours for a practiced judge, and more as the system is first being learned. Many judges find it useful to view a few cases; assign only tentative ratings and classifications; and assign the final classification only after thinking the case over for a day or two. This is not necessary for all cases, but is often helpful because of the extensive behavioral repertoire of the 6-year-old.

Order of Assessments

This is the suggested order for the use of the sixth-year attachment systems. Rating a particular 3-minute episode is expected to take from 1 to 2 hours. However, we suggest that you may not want to assign final ratings or classifications immediately upon your final review of the tape. Once you have stopped viewing the tape, you may want to think for some time further.

Raters new to these systems should review all systems, and then review tapes for at least 30 children in their sample. This will give a notion of range and variation in type. In general, practiced raters profit a great deal from making mental comparisons with other children in a given sample, and raters new to a system will be greatly disadvantaged without an initial review of the range of behavior patterns.

Here, we suggest the order of procedures for use of these systems.

Step I. Repeated Review of the First 6 Seconds of the Tape (30 seconds of reunion) to Form a Hypothesis

The video-tapes you are using should have been spliced together so that each episode begins 30 seconds before the parent's entrance. Before attempting the application of *any* system, review the first 60 seconds of your episode (30 seconds before, plus 30 second after, the parent's entrance), using slow motion.

DO NOT GO ANY FURTHER! Review in regular and slow motion alternately at least five and up to ten times, until you think you understand what the return of the parent "means" to this child (remember, you are beginning at the point just prior to the child's realization that the parent is about to enter). You have a chance to assess the child's mood prior to this realization; the child's response to recognition of the parent's coming entrance; and the first 30 seconds of response to the entrance itself.

The first contrast you will be able to make from this review is between the child who remains essentially calm at learning the parent is about to enter the room, and the child who undertakes a major change in her behavior. A child can be considered essentially calm if she smiles and shows some pleasure, tries to hide her pleasure in "reserve," makes no initial large changes in behavior, or looks up from her play and says "Well! At last you came back!" If, however, the child seems to you to "need" to do something about the return of the parent, and this need is manifested in a major change in behavior, this is your first index of potential insecurity. This child is changing its attentional and behavioral organization in order to deal with the return of the parent. It would seem to be a sign of insecurity if at the moment of entrance the child:

1. Stiffens, becomes more tense, or moves away.
2. Shows too bright or eager a response, for example, running to the door, saying "Gee! Wow! It's Mom!" followed by a flat expression or by avoidance.
3. Tries to keep the parent out of the room, suggests immediately that the parent does not enter or interrupt, or suggests that the parent goes away.
4. Gives a dismissing greeting ("HEL-lo"), or points immediately to some object which may distract the parent's attention from interaction.
5. Upon recognizing that the parent is about to enter, the child changes the object of her attention, suddenly becoming attentive to toys or objects which had not attracted her attention a moment previously.
6. Shows a sudden, nervous smile or nervous change in behavior, for example, ducking down behind something, dropping something, suddenly jumping up on something.

These are only examples: There will be many other patterns of behavior not suggested or described earlier. In general, continually review these 60 seconds until you feel you understand the child's response to the parent's re-entry. This means that you have developed a "hypothesis" which you can test further as you view the remainder of the episode.

This hypothesis may well be disconfirmed, but in forming it, you will become active in your participation in the further study of the child and parent.

Step II. "Mapping" the Episode

Now review the entire episode two or three times to map out what happens, and in what order. You need to be sure of exactly what is being said, who is being addressed, and who is moving where (and why) at this point in the procedure.

This map of the proceedings (and internal transcript of the speech) should be firmly in mind before you begin to review the tape for assessments in terms of specific systems.

Now play the tape through both quickly and slowly without sound. Are there any special movements or facial expressions on the part of the child, which were masked by the confusion of the movement and speech of several people – movements or expressions which are particularly indicative of security or insecurity, or which remain to be explained?

Step III. Rating for Avoidance

Review the full scale before starting to attempt to identify a particular area in which this child may fall. After reviewing the full scale, review the full tape twice.

Now begin reviewing the tape in conjunction with the rating system, utilizing slow motion, fast motion, etc. Review the tape once without sound, and once listening especially to the quality of the child's voice.

Consider the function served by avoidance as well as the specific identifiers.

Step IV. Rating for Security

Review the "security" scoring system – reading all points, not only those which seem likely following your preliminary review of the tape itself. Now begin reviewing the tape in conjunction with the rating system, utilizing slow motion, freezing, backing up, and re-reviewing until you feel you understand each behavioral sequence. This is an important assessment because it allows you to determine whether, for example, a child who is to be classified as insecure-avoidant is either very insecure (rated 9 on the 9-point scale) or only slightly insecure (6) overall.

Step V. Classification

This is the most difficult step. If you are satisfied with your ratings for security and avoidance, you will be somewhat advanced toward making the security classification. If you have scored the child from 5 to 9 on the scale, she should be classified as secure or as very secure. Scores from 1 to 3 mean that the child is insecure, while a score of 4 indicates that the child could be in your final judgment classified as either secure or insecure. The child is already classified as avoidant if she has been given scores from 6 to 7 on avoidance.

There are four major classifications, another "insecure-unclassified" classification, and a number of sub-classifications to be assigned. If the child is given either the insecure-directing or the insecure-unclassified classification, she must also be given an "A, B, C" classification and sub-classification. Also, if the child is assigned an A, B, or C classification with a "D" subscript, she must still be given a forced A, B, C sub-category.

Obviously, assigning the classification takes several more reviews of the tape. However, you may not feel ready to assign the classification immediately upon completing your review of the tape. You may want to simply think about the tape for several hours or even several days, before assigning the final classification.

Secure vs. Insecure Attachment: Rating Scale

This is a 9-point scale for rating the security vs. insecurity the child seems to experience in relationship to the parent (9 is high). Anchor points for the scale are listed below. Scores of 2, 4, 6, and 8 are, of course, given as frequently as those for which scale-points are defined. Some raters use half-points, for example, 5.5.

Score 9 – Very Secure. Either the child initiates proximity and contact of an unambivalent and affectionate nature during the episode, or the child initiates real and personal contact with respect to conversation. These initiations are often accompanied by a "full" look into the parent's face in the first moments of reunion.

A child qualifies for this highest rating only if she initiates a direct and full-faced look into the parent's face, aligning her face to look as fully as possible into that of the parent in the first moments of reunion. If this look does not have the "forced," deliberate quality of the over-bright greeting, it is one of the primary indices of strong security. The look is usually faintly lingering.

Physical contact in a very secure child often looks casual. The child may rest a hand casually upon the parent's knee in the course of doing something else; lie momentarily across a seated parent's legs when reaching for a toy; or touch the parent when passing by in a crowded corner. (Note: Children occasionally initiate proximity or contact which cannot be termed affectionate, or which is not maintained once initiated. If a child initiates proximity aggressively, or while making aggressive remarks, it is not the initiation of a secure child. This is likewise the case for sexual initiations, as well as for contact, which is suddenly broken or treated as though it were uncomfortable).

Verbal initiation may take several forms. For example, the child may invite the parent to play or to join in play; take a personal interest in the parent's own activities; or may be eager to explain what she has been doing or playing with. Note again, for the highest rating, the child is actively initiating of positive interaction or of affectionate moves into increased proximity or (even if casual) contact.

Although initiating, the very secure child is relaxed, confident, and calm. The child is pleased at the parent's return but neither surprised by it nor overly eager, bright, or caregiving. There is no sudden, major re-organization in the child's behavior.

Score 7 – Secure. The child is clearly at ease with the parent, clearly pleased about the parent's return (although perhaps trying to cover it up a bit with reserve or "feistiness"). Although this child does not initiate contact or interaction, she is clearly ready to communicate and interact with the parent, and she is definitely responsive to parental initiations.

Responsiveness may be shown by ready, eager expansion of the parent's own remarks. That is, the child's responses to the parent may serve to continue, prolong, or expand the conversation. For instance, if the parent says, "That castle is like Michael's," and the child responds, "Yeah, it is. Only his is a little bigger, and red. Did you see all these guys with funny hats in the castle?", then an expansion is noted. The child makes clear with responses such as this that conversation and dialogue are welcomed.

Responsiveness may also be shown by the child's breaking in eagerly to add her own thoughts, observations, comments, or (not unpleasant) contradictions while the parent is speaking. The speech quality between parent and child is comfortable.

Score 5 – Probably Secure. The child is given this rating when the "best guess" is that the child is secure with the parent. This rating is given if (a) the child shows no marked signs of either security or insecurity but seems sufficiently at ease and without anxiety in the presence of the parent to be given this rating, or if (b) the child shows some signs of security sufficient for a higher rating, but some difficulty is exhibited which lowers the ratings. For example, the child's reserve lasts too long, although then the child is responsive.

Score 3 – Insecure. The child is neutrally avoidant, is directing-caregiving, is moderately ambivalent, etc. The child will definitely be placed in one of the insecure classifications, but, there are still some signs of a remaining confidence in the relationship.

Score 1 – Very Insecure. The child is extremely avoidant, extremely punitive, extremely ambivalent, or shows several combined signs of insecurity. Either the strategies used to deal with the parent are extreme in themselves (suggesting extreme insecurity in the relationship), or several are combined (suggesting strong insecurity, but no single strategy for dealing with it). No signs of real security or confidence in the parent are present. (See the section on classification for a detailed description of behaviors characterizing insecure attachments at 6 years of age).

Note: Children assigned a 7 or above for security or confidence are almost always assigned to the B3-equivalent classification. Children assigned a 5 or a 6 are almost always assigned to one of the other "B" classifications. Children given a rating between 1 and 3 points on this scale are assigned to one of the insecure classifications. A rating of 4 may be given to children who will ultimately be assigned to either the secure or the several insecure classifications. Conversely, children who are classified A, C, D, or O may have received any rating between 1 and 4 on the security scale.

Avoidance of Proximity and Emotional Interaction

This scoring system deals with the intensity, persistence, duration, and promptness of the child's avoidance of physical or personal interaction, proximity, or contact. Avoidant behaviors may be defined as any behaviors which function to maintain or to increase the physical or affective and emotional distance between the child and parent, through a shift of attention away from the parent, or through preserving attention to other occupations, conversations, or objects.

The critical moments for avoidance are those for which acknowledgment of intimacy of relationship is most expected. Thus, the first moments of reunion after a substantial separation, as well as any moment at which the parent requests the child's attention are moments of special importance.

A highly avoidant child may initiate certain types of proximity-seeking or interaction when the parent's attention is focused elsewhere, or at moments when proximity and interaction are not expected. Acknowledgment of the relationship at the moment of reunion, and at moments when the parent seeks acknowledgment, is, however, avoided. At such moments, the child may be at special risk for displaying affection, distress, or anger and hence may seek to maintain a distance through avoidance.

What behaviors are considered avoidant? A partial list includes: moving away from the parent on reunion; keeping the back turned or actively turning the back to the parent on reunion; seeming pre-occupied with toys or persons other than the parent, while the body is kept slightly aligned away from the parent; ignoring the parent's overtures while looking otherwise pre-occupied; responding to overtures whenever necessary, but as minimally as possible; and attempting to distract the parent's attention to things other than the child herself. As the reader will infer from this list, *the tone of avoidance is neutral.* Both affection and anger are absent.

Contra-indications for avoidance include proximity-seeking or verbal initiations, which are genuinely affectionate or relationship-acknowledging; eager responsiveness in conversation; full, open looks into the parent's face; and annoyance, anger, or punitiveness, however expressed.

Because avoidance is neutral rather than either affectionate or confrontational in style, the strategies needed to maintain neutrality will depend upon the reunion behavior of the parent. If the parent, as well as child, fails to acknowledge reunion, the highly avoidant child can maintain distance from the parent through silence, failure to greet, and failure to initiate. But if a parent presses hard or repeatedly, a 6-year-old child who wishes to maintain distance in order to avoid emotional interaction needs to give some minimal replies. The 6-year-old, in contrast to the 1-year-old, is likely aware that failure to respond when pressed risks *increasing* parental attention, and hence creating an emotionally tinged confrontation. In such a circumstance, the child may not only reply, but may also initiate proximity or conversation, which is neutral in topic or tone. A highly avoidant child, in contrast to a punitive or confrontational child, is willing to respond, as seems necessary to maintain emotional distance, and may even greet the parent with the apparent purpose of getting past the social niceties. *A highly avoidant child ignores the parent's initiations only so long as it is possible to do this while appearing neutral and/or otherwise occupied.*

Because the function of avoidance is to avoid affectively tinged interchange, a highly avoidant child will appear merely busy while ignoring the parent, and in interaction will appear neutral or polite. Even in moving away from the parent soon following the reunion, the child will appear not really to be moving away from the parent but rather to be moving toward something else. Thus, the child appears to need to fetch an object for further play in the sandbox, or merely to want to return immediately to play already established. Similarly, in turning away or remaining turned away, the child seems to be getting something or playing with something. Not to have such a rationale for moving away or staying away from the parent would be to risk confrontation. A highly avoidant child does not really want the parent to ask what she is doing or why.

Avoidance is scored on a 1–7 point scale, where 1 indicates no avoidance, and 7 indicates strong avoidance. Before moving to the actual directions for rating, you should read the following three sections:

Indications of avoidance. This section lists behaviors considered both moderately and strongly avoidant. It also stresses the importance of context in judging avoidance at 6 years of age. In certain contexts, not speaking to the parent when spoken to is avoidant, while in others, it is punitive or confrontational. In certain contexts, not-looking is avoidant, whereas in others it seems to signal feelings of hurt or anger, and as such is only minimally avoidant.

Forms of proximity-seeking, greeting, and speech consonant with strong avoidance. The highly avoidant child may occasionally greet the parent, approach the parent, or speak with the parent. In this section, types of greeting, speech, and proximity-seeking which are consonant with the maintenance of emotional distance between parent and child are listed. Each of these can appear in a child who shows strong avoidance, without reducing the rating for avoidance.

Forms of greeting, speech, and proximity-seeking inconsonant with high scores for avoidance. Genuinely affectionate, openly angry, and any other relationship-acknowledging behavior is inconsonant with high avoidance. If it appears *following* moderate to strong avoidance, it represents a breakdown of avoidance, and high scores can no longer be given. Similarly, high scores cannot be given if the child, while keeping her back turned much of the time, either strongly expresses anger or turns toward the parent for frequent looks and smiles. Judges score an episode by first looking for indications of avoidance, and then seeing whether greeting, speech, or proximity-seeking is of a type to reduce the score otherwise given for avoidance.

Indications of Avoidance

The moment of reunion is a moment when re-establishment or affirmation of relationship is most expected or called for. Strong avoidance at this moment indicates that the child is unable or unwilling to acknowledge or affirm the relationship. A child can maintain or increase the distance between herself and the parent through several means: physical avoidance, visual avoidance, and avoidance of conversational response.

At 12–18 months of age, these three behaviors – moving away from the parent, averting the gaze from the parent, and not responding when addressed – are all considered avoidant behaviors. Yet by 6 years, behavioral meaning has changed. At six, almost all physical movements away can still be considered avoidant. By six, however, failing to look and failing to speak can serve an emotionally communicative function rather than an avoidant one. By this age, the child has frequently learned the unwritten social rules. At times, not-looking is not avoidant so much as it is communicative of hurt or hostility (as is not-speaking). At other times, not-looking and not-speaking are still efforts to avoid communication. Moving away from the parent on reunion, which is almost always considered avoidant, is discussed first here. The importance of context in visual avoidance and conversational avoidance is then discussed.

Physical Avoidance

Physical avoidance includes moving away, orienting or remaining oriented away, and aligning the body away from the parent. What is it that the child is avoiding? The child seems to be avoiding not only proximity and contact but also any orientation, which would make communication – especially, affectively tinged communication – more likely.

Physical closeness and body alignment are not only communicative in themselves, but they also increase the likelihood of mutual attention and communication. Ventral–ventral contact or even ventral–ventral orientation across a distance is especially likely to be avoided.

If a child shows *any* of the following behaviors at the moment of reunion, the child will receive a very high rating for avoidance, *unless* there is strongly affectionate or angry initiation or responsiveness later in the episode.

a. Moving away from the parent almost immediately upon reunion, that is, just following an initial greeting. (Be careful here. Most avoidant children will appear to be getting a toy, and all will have some rationale. Moving away is meaningful in itself. Even if a child merely immediately moves away to get something to bring back to the parent, the move away is slightly avoidant.) A move away in which the child remains at a distance is highly avoidant.
b. Turning the back to the parent upon reunion, and staying with the back to the parent for more than 5 seconds.
c. Keeping the back oriented to the parent on reunion, that is, not turning about to look at the parent, or looking only very briefly about, as though out of curiosity. This is given a high score if the child remains with back turned more than 5 seconds. (Note: Remaining oriented away from the parent is

not a movement, but nonetheless it is highly avoidant. It indicates the child is busy; it indicates that this is not a special moment; and it leaves the child in a position from which little further communication can be expected).

d. Moving forward to greet the parent, then dashing away from the parent with the back to the parent, and usually forward into the room. Here the child seems to have attempted to greet the parent, then suddenly to have had to turn away and move away with the back to the parent. Again, because the avoidant child always looks neutral and seems to have a rationale, the child in this circumstance usually looks as though she is merely leading the parent into the room, going back to play, or going to interact with the other parent. Nonetheless, such a strong move away indicates a strong difficulty acknowledging the relationship, and hence is avoidant.

All the above behaviors yield high scores for avoidance only when they occur immediately upon reunion. A minute or so following a full greeting, moving away to play or to speak with the other parent may not be at all avoidant.

Other physical movements or orientations, which should yield *some* score for avoidance are:

a. Keeping the body or head angled away from the parent, keeping the shoulder interposed between self and parent, etc.
b. Breaking contact with the parent, no matter who initiated the contact.
c. Showing an aversion to ventral orientation or contact with the parent, even when in bodily contact with the parent.
d. Attempting, immediately upon reunion, to orient the parent's attention away from the child, for example, "Look at that toy over there." This is an avoidant behavior, because it attempts to re-direct the parent's attention or orientation elsewhere, hence to avoid mutuality.

Visual Avoidance – Averting the Gaze

At six, not-looking is still considered avoidant behavior if: The child distinctly aligns the head or body away from the parent and toward some other object of attention (toys, other parent, mirrors, etc.). Thus, if the child is not-looking because of being busily bent over the sandbox, talking with the examiner, or if the child is aligning the head so that the child could not see the parent without a major change in posture, the not-looking is avoidant. This is because with this type of visual avoidance, the child seems to try to indicate that he is too busy to interact just now, not a suitable candidate for attention, etc.

At six, not-looking is especially likely to be a meta-signal for hurt or anger, and hence only minimally avoidant, if:

a. The child has a fairly open physical orientation to the parent.
b. The child is interacting, initiating, or being at least moderately responsive, whether pleasantly or unpleasantly. If a child looks down or seems muted

while interacting either pleasantly or unpleasantly with the parent, the child seems to be adding a meta-communication to the present communication such as, ". . . and I'm a bit hurt or puzzled, so you might want to ask me about it," or, ". . . I'm not only feeling nasty enough to speak to you the way I'm speaking to you, but you can't make me look at you either."

So, a muted not-looking *while interacting* (or in the context of being interactive frequently during the episode) is not really avoidant. As a rule of thumb, add only 1 point to what would otherwise be the child's score for avoidance.

Conversational Avoidance: Not-Speaking and "Minimizing" Responses

To begin with, at six, there are general qualities of response or initiation in speech, which are indicative of avoidance. These include:

a. Flat tones in speech.
b. Dismissing tones in greeting.
c. Minimal responses to questions and statements from the parent. These minimal responses can be safely used by a highly avoidant child because they do not increase the likelihood of further conversation, yet they are satisfactory enough that they do not attract increased attention from the parent. As an example, the parent may ask, "So, you've been playing all this time with Carol?", and the child may answer "Yeah," or the parent may ask, "So, what have you been playing with?", and the child may answer, "The truck."

The general sense gained from these qualities of speech is that the child is busy or pre-occupied, but willing to get through the social niceties while not encouraging further conversation.

When the child is directly addressed by the parent and does not reply, not-speaking can be either avoidant or communicative. At six, not-speaking when addressed is still avoidant rather than communicative if:

a. It is accompanied by efforts to look busy or as though it was not possible to hear the parent.
b. It occurs at a point where the parent could be, or was, interacting with someone else anyway, and only addressed the child casually.
c. It occurs when the child has her back to the parent, or is markedly oriented away from the parent, which would already indicate that attention is elsewhere.

In general, *not-speaking is avoidant if it could go unnoticed,* or if the child may think it could go unnoticed, or if the parent could reasonably think the child did not hear, did not notice, or was merely pre-occupied. Thus, silence or ignoring in these contexts is discouraging of further efforts on the part of the parent, but is not confrontational. The child's failure to respond communicates, "I really am busy/am thinking of something else/didn't notice what you said/didn't hear you."

At six, not-speaking when addressed is *punitive and confrontational rather than avoidant* if it seems to function to humiliate, hurt, or embarrass the parent. This is the case when:

a. The parent is in a position to easily see the child's face, the child refuses to respond or speak, and the child does not bother to orient away from the parent to "cover" for this failure of response.
b. The parent is speaking in a manner, which betrays a "need" for the child to respond vocally. For example, the parent addresses the child repeatedly, without answer from the child. The embarrassing or even humiliating apparent intent of this behavior was particularly striking in our Berkeley study, where the child behaved in this way "in front of" the examiner.
c. The parent is greeting the child – a moment that the child knows by age six to be especially sensitive.

Forms of Greeting, Speech, and Proximity-Seeking CONSONANT with Strong Avoidance

Children receiving the highest scores for avoidance may nonetheless greet the parent (either in response or in initiation), respond when addressed, initiate certain types of conversation, or approach the parent for certain purposes.

In many or most cases, these initiations or responses seem to maintain the interactive distance between child and parent. In some cases, it seems clear that they are, in fact, *necessary* if distance is to be maintained.

Greetings Consonant with Strong Avoidance

Greeting, smiling, and showing the parent something may be seen in avoidant children who seem to need to get past the social niceties in order to maintain social distance and to avoid further, possibly emotional, interchange. Watch carefully for signs that an apparent greeting is actually avoidant of continuing or opening communication. Watch here for a flat or dismissing tone of voice, or a limited or "false" smile. At the moment of reunion, the avoidant child may show the parent a toy in a way which distracts the parent's attention from the child. This is contrasted with showing off of something the child has done or accomplished, a behavior which would lead to further personal contact.

Speech consonant with strong avoidance.

Initiations or responses which:

a. Are simply neutral or business-like, and do not suggest a need for further affective interchange between child and parent (essentially, which are "rhetorical"). As an example, the child responds with "Yeah, I drew the family," "Nope," "The truck," "Uh-huh," "I need a pencil."

b. Are help-seeking or help-offering when the tone is polite or neutral, as to a neighbor or teacher. As an example, the child says, "Fix my buttons," "I can find it," "You can get at it from here."
c. Occur in response to the parent's repeated pressing of the child for information. The avoidant child who is repeatedly or strongly pressed by the parent has to make some acknowledgment, and may do so by giving minimal repeated "yes" or "no" answers, or giggling self-consciously without looking at the parent (seen twice in girls attempting to "avoid" a particularly pressing father), or even by trying to make some sort of initiation. This repeated pressing necessitates some response in order to maintain distance.
d. Are odd in content, senseless, pointless, or strange. In addition, conversation with content which is, in a *neutral* way, threatening or aggressive. Neutrally aggressive speech neither encourages interaction nor brooks emotional response from the parent. Examples: "Eeech, eech, eech!", or "Tigers, tigers, tigers gonna throw you up!", or "You're gonna be sick, so sick" (said in an odd, affectless sing-song, directed to no one). This speech is not directly angry or confrontational; hence, it does not reduce a score otherwise given for avoidance.

Proximity-seeking consonant with strong avoidance.

a. Proximity-seeking or contact-seeking which is business-like in purpose (help-seeking, for example, fixing the child's buttons, or help-offering, for example, showing the parent politely the way to the bathroom); odd in purpose; or aggressive in purpose.
b. Proximity-seeking immediately upon reunion, which is followed immediately by dashing away from the parent and forward into the room, toward a toy or other person, etc. The initial movement toward the parent may be one of intended greeting – but if this is followed immediately by a move away, a strong score for avoidance may well be given.

Forms of Greeting, Speech, and Proximity-Seeking INCONSONANT with High Scores for Avoidance

In general, any greeting, pattern of speech or proximity-seeking which is intimate, emotional, or confrontational is inconsonant with high scores for avoidance.

Greeting

"Secure" or genuinely positive greetings, which are an immediate, full acknowledgment of the parent's return, and hence subtly recognizing the importance of the parent's absence.

Examples include:

a. Full, genuine greeting and look of pleasure or delight.
b. Deliberate craning about to look fully into the parent's face.
c. Immediate remark acknowledging the separation, such as, "Mom, guess what we did while you were gone?" (Compare this to an at least potentially avoidant greeting of, "Look at the toy horse," which does not recognize absence, reunion, or relationship).
d. "Insecure" or negative responses to reunion which are rejecting of the parent, humiliating to the parent, or embarrassing to the parent, and hence confrontational. Here too the relationship is immediately recognized and called upon, even though the expression may be punitive silence or overt rejection.

Speech.
Conversational *initiations* such as the following:

a. Inviting parent to play with or join child.
b. Showing interest in the parent's own activities.
c. Making a supportive remark to or about the parent.
d. Making a personal remark about her own state or that of the parent, positive *or* negative ("I'm really tired," and "You are a big bore" are both personal and non-avoidant).
e. Initiating a new topic of conversation, which can be readily expanded upon by the parent, such as, "I made a castle just like the one we have at home, remember?"
f. Making an openly angry, rejecting, or humiliating remark to the parent.

Conversational responsiveness with the following characteristics:

a. Quick responses to the parent's speech, as though eager, or at least very familiar and ready. This may be, again, either positive or negative.
b. Eager interruptions of the parent's speech for the purpose of communication (interrupt to answer, to ask questions, to tell of own activities).
c. Fuller responses to parent's speech or questions than is necessary (expansions). In response to "Did you make that?", the child says not merely "Yes," but, "Yes, I made that one and this one too. I'm an architect!"
d. Expanding on conversation or questions. "Yes, and I made this and this too. Actually, you oughta see the blue one. I made it first."

Proximity-Seeking

Any form of affectionate contact, whether direct or having a familiar casualness, is inconsonant with high scores for avoidance. (But see forms of proximity-seeking which are not inconsonant with strong avoidance, such as those which are subtly aggressive, threatening, or uncomfortable, or proximity-seeking which is followed immediately by a dash ahead of or away from the parent).

Avoidance Rating System

The original system for scoring avoidance was devised by Ainsworth for use with 12-month-old infants in a situation in which the behavior of the mother was substantially controlled. Her scoring system described over 20 exact behavior patterns, with some modifications for the mother's pressing or not pressing the infant for interaction.

Because Ainsworth could identify most of the possible "avoidant" patterns, which would be seen in the repertoire of the 1-year-old, her system was justifiably called a scoring rather than a rating system. Thus, each major pattern of response was listed, and judges identified the pattern and gave the score for avoidance only afterwards.

The present system is devised for use with 6-year-old children in a situation in which the behavior of the parent is completely uncontrolled. Moreover, the situation is complex socially, in that the adult examiner does not leave the room on the parent's return, and (in the Berkeley laboratory) the second parent returns to the child, the examiner, and the first parent. Finally, the repertoire of the 6-year-old is almost as complex socially as the repertoire of the adult, and the 6-year-old can use language to avoid, or to re-direct the parent's attention.

This given, it is not possible to devise a scoring system which will give the judge the full repertoire of behavior patterns. We suggest training on an initial sample of 15 reunions, which represent the full range of avoidance (from none, to the highest score of 7). The judge should be thoroughly familiar with all parts of this avoidance-scoring manual, and should review it frequently.

In scoring a reunion, the procedure is as follows:

a. Review the section of this manual entitled "Indications of Avoidance," and note any which are present on the tape.
b. No child is avoidant throughout an entire reunion episode unless the parent is completely cooperative in maintaining the avoidance, and does not address the child nor approach her. Therefore, examine all greeting, speech, and proximity-seeking carefully, using the relevant parts of this manual to determine whether it is of a form consonant or inconsonant with high scores for avoidance.
c. This rating system is a final guideline, but it is necessarily limited. Children may show combinations of behavior not listed here. Your overall sense of the degree of avoidance relative to other children in the same sample is also a guideline to the rating given for avoidance.

Scale for Rating Avoidance

Avoidance is scored on a 7-point scale for comparison with the Ainsworth system. A score of one is given if the child shows no avoidance, a score of 7 if the child shows very strong avoidance.

A score of "1" can be given if:

a. The child greets the parent with delight, and easy interchanges follow. Occasionally, the child looks away or is occupied with other things, but this happens only after the relationship is clearly re-established.
b. The child greets the parent or responds to the parent, but without ardor or special delight. Soon after reunion, the child either looks into the parent's face lingeringly or fully, or verbally re-affirms the special nature of the relationship. These signs of readiness for communication may follow a casual greeting, but in their fullness, they are meaningful even though they are not accompanied by smiles.
c. The child greets the parent with hostility or rejection, and is directing or cruel during the episode. There is no physical avoidance, however, and the child seems to look at the parent readily. The response to the parent is immediate and not casual.
d. Note that following a full greeting, a return to play, or a turn to conversing with the other parent or with the examiner is not considered to be avoidance of the parent.

Score "1.5 to 3.5" for brief but limited, or persistent but faint, avoidance:

a. The child is largely responsive and interactive but fails to look at the parent while responding and interacting as much as would be expected (low score).
b. Brief avoidance of the parent, as in not-looking or a delay in reply, followed by responsiveness and initiations – but, the child does not look at the parent as much as would be expected.
c. Hostile responses to the parent, followed by continuing hostility or punitiveness while looking down or refusing to meet the gaze of the parent.
d. The child gives a genuinely positive greeting, but this is followed by some active avoidance or avoidantly casual interaction, or by an "avoidant" response to contact with the parent.
e. Sharp immediate avoidance which is followed by real responsiveness or by initiations of contact of a genuinely affectionate (or even caregiving) nature. The score here depends on the degree to which the child warms up to, or even takes the initiative with the parent through behaviors inconsonant with high scores for avoidance.
f. Brief period of ignoring the parent followed by regaining of responsiveness or by making initiations to the parent.
g. The child is slow to look at the parent or to respond to her overtures – but then she does respond. However, while she acknowledges and responds to the parent's overtures, she is muted and is not initiating (higher end).

h. The child greets the parent, and then shows some slight reserve. She is then responsive either in interacting with the parent or in exchanging looks, smiles, and conversation in the course of play. She does not, however, take the initiative in seeking interaction and contact.
i. The child's initial avoidance is very slight, but there is a mutedness accompanying responsiveness throughout the episode. The eyes are downcast, or the child is a little slow to respond (as though she is faintly hurt or puzzled), but generally she seems at ease with the parent (low score).

Score between "4 and 5" if the child shows brief but strong avoidance, or a persistent low-keyed avoidance (seeming too casual).

a. Strong avoidance followed by some real responsiveness (friendly or hostile) which is nonetheless slightly limited.
b. The child greets her parent (positively or negatively) and may start to approach her but then shows some avoidance. The child continues with her play, or conversation, perhaps with occasional looks, smiles, or interchanges with the parent. What is avoidant here is the failure to "recognize" the separation in the excessive casualness of the interchange upon reunion.
c. The child fails to greet the parent and ignores the parent most of the time, keeping busy with other things. However, there are flashes of some directness, whether of rejection or warmth, and these flashes show an underlying relatedness. The child does not really "warm-up" to the parent over the episode, however. There is no flow of responsiveness and no real initiation.
d. The child ignores the parent at first, then responds, but without much elaboration. The child's behavior may be "difficult," or even faintly punitive, but perhaps because of this there seems to be a parent–child connection. A striking element may again be casualness, as though nothing had happened.

Score "5.5 to 7" whenever the child seems extremely neutral, or organized, or rigid with respect to the parent.

High scores are given when it seems unlikely that the child could easily break through avoidance to expressions of anger, affection, or hurt and distress. They can be given even when the child gives a flat initiating greeting, and even when the child seeks proximity for certain purposes (as, to politely show the parent the way to the bathroom, as though the parent were a neighbor or teacher).

Scores above 5.5 cannot be given if the child shows clear annoyance, clear pleasure, or hurt during the episode. Nor can they be given if there is affectionate contact-seeking, or initiations of personal or inviting conversation.

a. The child keeps her back to the parent for longer than 5 seconds following the parent's entrance. There is a definite rigidity or stiffness. The child may then break this rigid orientation with an initiation of a neutral type; or may converse with her back to the parent; or may remain oriented away even when the parent approaches or touches, then make a "necessary" response or initiation of a type consonant with strong avoidance (highest score for this last pattern).

b. There is an approach followed immediately by withdrawal. This is usually seen as dashing into the room ahead of the parent, back to a toy or to the other parent, etc. After this, interaction has a neutral quality.
c. The reunion looks neutral, innocuous, affectless, and unimportant. The child may "greet" the parent, observing the niceties. After that, the parent does not press for interaction, and the child remains otherwise occupied, without speaking to the parent for all or most of the episode.
d. The child attempts to ignore or avoid the parent on reunion, but the parent presses continually for interaction. The child gives minimal acknowledgments, in the forms of words or perhaps of little giggles, but there is no initiation on the part of the child and no responsiveness other than what the parent has made necessary.

Attachment Classifications for 6-Year-Olds

This is a set of classifications and sub-classifications describing major differences in the organization of a child's attachment to the parent at 6 years of age. The major classifications correspond to the major classifications discovered to date in infancy: secure (group B), insecure-avoidant (group A), insecure-ambivalent (group C), and insecure-disorganized (identified as group D in infancy, but as insecure-directing at 6 years of age). There are sub-classifications within the major categories. In addition, a child may be insecure-unclassified (group O). A child who is determined to be insecure-directing or to be insecure-unclassified is always given a "best-fitting" or "forced" A, B, or C classification.

A picture of the classification system is drawn as follows in Table 7.1. In the first column the equivalent status in infancy is described, for example, the Controlling/Directing 6-year-old is expected to have been insecure-disorganized. The second column gives the sixth-year category title. The third title informs the reader whether an alternative, "forced" A, B, C classification needs to be assigned. Thus, for every 6-year-old determined to be secure with some resemblance to the controlling/directing or unclassified child, a best-fitting "Ainsworth" sub-group must still be assigned.

A judge who is new to this system should first review the scale for rating security, the scale for rating avoidance, and this classification system thoroughly. She or he should then review at least 30 cases in the sample to be judged, to acquire a sense of the range of behavior within that sample. Children who have been rated between 5 and 9 on the security rating scale automatically are placed in one of the secure categories, while children rated from 1 to 3 are automatically placed in one of the three insecure categories.

Table 7.1 Attachment classification system

Infancy Equivalent	*Sixth-Year Class*	*"Forced Class"*
Group B (Secure)	*Secure (B)*	
B1	Secure-reserved (B1) but verbally playful	Not necessary
B2	Secure-reserved (B2)	Not necessary
B3	Very secure (B3)	Not necessary
B4	Secure-feisty (B4a) Secure-immature (B4b) Secure-disorganized (B4c)	Not necessary
B(D)	Secure – resembles Controlling or Unclassified	Assign B1, B2, B3, B4
Group A (Avoidant)	*Avoidant*	
A1	Extremely avoidant (A1)	Not necessary
A2	Neutral-avoidant (A2)	Not necessary
A(D)	Avoidant-resembles Controlling or Unclassified	Assign A1 or A2
Group C (Ambivalent)	*Ambivalent*	
C1	Hostile (C1)	Not necessary
C2	Passive (C2)	Not necessary
C(D)	Ambivalent-resembles Controlling or Unclassified	Assign C1 or C2
Group D (Disorganized)	*Controlling (Directing)*	
No sub-groups	Controlling-punitive (D1)	Necessary
	Controlling-caregiving (D2)	Not necessary
	– caregiving/guiding (D2a)	Not necessary
	– over-bright/cheering (D2b)	Not necessary
Other	*Insecure-unclassified*	
Example: Not attached	Example: Sexualized, or insecure-can't classify	Necessary

The rating of 4 yields an ultimate assignment of either a secure or an insecure category. Classification is the last step in the analysis of any reunion episode.

Secure (Group B): Confident in the Relationship

Children are judged secure in the relationship to the parent at 6 years of age when they show some genuine *pleasure* in the parent and/or at the parent's return; and when they seem essentially *relaxed* (*calm*) throughout the episode (although they may be somewhat reserved or somewhat high-spirited, or "feisty"). These children may initiate interaction, proximity, or contact with the parent, or may simply be genuinely responsive to the parent's own initiations. If there are signs of some insecurity, they are overridden by an essential confidence.

VERY SECURE

Either the child initiates proximity and contact of an unambivalent and affectionate nature during the episode; or the child initiates real and personal contact with respect to conversation; or, the child is *highly* responsive to parental initiations.

A very secure child *often initiates a particularly direct and full-faced look into the parent's face, aligning her face to look as fully as possible into that of the parent.* Re-alignment of the body in order to gaze fully into the parent's face immediately upon entrance is a strong sign of security. The look is usually faintly lingering.

SECURE-RESERVED (B1 AND/OR B2)

In an essentially secure child, some reserve may be shown at the parent's entrance, but it is short-lived and seems to serve one of two purposes: It may serve as a "cover-up" for caring or pleasure, as in the case of the 6-year-old who grins broadly when he realizes that the parent is returning, then tries to look serious, straight-faced, and busy when the parent actually enters. The child spends a few moments in studied casualness.

It may be that the child needs a moment to re-organize or re-accept the parent, to "realize" the parent is back and respond to her/him. This child may need a few moments before feeling can be shown, or a moment to re-organize and shift attention. The reserve shown here is not a strong avoidance, that is, it is not a moving away from the parent or a steady maintenance of an "away" orientation. These children behave like Ainsworth's secure-avoidant (B1 or B2) infants.

We are at present differentiating between children who are simply reserved (B2) and children who may be somewhat more physically avoidant and who in addition seem to use playful dialogue with the parent to express their underlying affection (B1). These parallels are deliberately drawn to the Ainsworth infancy classifications, in which the B1 infant substitutes interaction across a distance for proximity-seeking at the time of the parent's return.

SECURE-DEPENDENT (IMMATURE), "FEISTY," OR SLIGHTLY DISORGANIZED

In infancy, children are placed in this "secure" sub-category when they (meet the general descriptors for the "secure" category but also) focus their attention upon the mother through much of the Strange Situation, responding strongly to separation and perhaps taking somewhat longer to be settled than infants in the remaining "B" sub-categories. These children may show some resistance to the parent as well and in general bear some resemblance to both "C" and "D" infants during the Strange Situation.

The principle of organization of attachment relationship for these infants seems to be an exaggeration of dependence upon the parent. For these infants as seen during the Strange Situation, attachment-related emotions are emphasized over exploration, and the attachment relationship with the parent takes easy precedence over exploration. We found in the first Berkeley study that 6-year-olds who had been classified B4 as infants showed one of three patterns of reunion behavior: A high-spirited "feistiness" toward the parent, a slight disorganization at entrance that was soon recaptured, and more directly, exaggeration of dependence and immaturity. We see the disorganization as a direct sequel to the slight disorganization occasionally observed in B4 infants during the Strange Situation. Whereas in "D" infants the pattern appears as transformed into controlling behavior, in a few children it may be observed directly again upon reunion at 6 years of age. We see expressions of dependency – as, sitting comfortably on mother's lap for most of the reunion – and "feistiness"– as, spunkily back-talking the mother – as two sides of the same coin. The child who is being "feisty" shows off and exaggerates the importance of the relationship.

These behavior patterns may appear as combined, or, only one might appear during a given reunion episode:

Secure-feisty (B4). By this we mean a high-spiritedness, a spunkiness, or even a good-natured and confident bossiness. This can take the form of ordering the parent about (fondly, not punitively, e.g., "Mommy, come here and feel this sand!"), protesting the parent's maneuvers, for example, "NO daddy, that's MY castle, we're playing Separate Castles"; or confidently sticking up for oneself, for example, "No, I didn't either!"

A child may seem feisty when she is simply expressing herself or her wishes to a parent who may or may not concede to these and who retains the upper hand in the relationship. The child may be expressing genuine irritation or annoyance ("NO, daddy!"), but if so this is done with warmth and confidence.

This behavior sometimes seems to function to permit the child to "show off" the relationship or her confidence in it. It may seem as though the child is attempting to accomplish this through faint testing or teasing regarding the relationship. Perhaps the child seems to be attempting to demonstrate that the parent is responsive to her.

Secure-slightly disorganized (B4). The parent's entrance seems slightly disorganizing to the child, who may briefly appear sad, confused, or "fumbling for something to do" – as though the parent's entrance had brought with it a disturbing memory or element. Like the initially reserved child, however, this child soon moves from this state to one of essential confidence. (The initial disorganization is not extreme, but may appear in a facial expression, initial slight stumbling in speech, or fumbling in movement.)

Secure-immature/dependent (B4). The child is essentially secure but seems a little young for age. Without at all seeming to qualify for the ambivalent-passive (C2) category, the child seems young for age or seems to require more than usual degrees of physical contact with the parent.

Secure-resembles directing child (B(d)). This category was logically expectable, and some candidates for the category have emerged in conjunction with Cassidy's Charlottesville sample and with Main's new Berkeley sample. These are children who meet the general criteria for the secure category, but whose reunion behavior bears some resemblance to that of children in any of the "D" and "O" categories. Some of these children seem for whatever reason to be "acting out" in the presence of or toward the mother. At first glance, this could lead to placement in the "D" category, but their reunion behavior is not really insecure. On close examination, they are seen as simply *disobedient* rather than punitive or humiliating. Some of these children seem instead to be cheering, bright in mood, or slightly caregiving, toward the parent. However, they will be assigned instead to the B(d) category if (a) their behavior generally qualifies for placement in the B category and (b) there is reason to think they are simply tired, or responding to mother's mood of the moment. Children who seem essentially secure but slightly depressed should also be placed in this category.

These children cannot be classified as "D" because their disobedient behavior is not punitive or humiliating, and their caregiving behavior does not extend to role-reversal and does not seem to reflect their own anxiety. The category is logically expectable because in infancy, some "D" qualities (see as the precursors to insecure-directing) are frequently present on reunion but are insufficient to qualify the infant for the disorganized/disoriented category.

Insecure-Avoidant (Group A)

In a subtle and non-confrontational manner, the child avoids the parent. The child may either move away from the parent, or simply remain oriented away from the parent, and/or the child may non-confrontationally ignore the parent's presence and utterances.

When the child ignores or moves away from the parent, it is with an excuse or rationale of being otherwise engaged (occupied with the toys, looking for a toy, responding instead to the examiner). The tone of the behavior is neutral, not confrontational. The parent may be dealt with as a child deals with a teacher or neighbor with whom she is willing to exchange social niceties. Speech may sound flat or have a dismissing quality.

Full acquaintance with the scale for rating avoidance is, of course, most useful in making these classifications. If a child receives scores of 5.5 or higher for avoidance, the child will inevitably be placed in one of the avoidant categories. (Note here, as in the avoidance rating system, that a child who dashes to greet the parent, then turns and immediately dashes away in an avoidant manner, can still be given a high rating for avoidance. Similarly, such a child can still be placed in the avoidant category).

Two sub-classifications may be distinguished:

Highly avoidant (A1). The child seems affectless with regard to the parent during interaction, and either actively moves away from the parent, or stays oriented away from the parent. Often, the child moves to a greater physical distance from the parent upon the parent's entrance. This is done subtly: The child appears to have a "rationale" (e.g., a toy of interest at a greater distance from the parent). The child may speak whenever spoken to, but topics remain neutral and impersonal. The child does not warm to the parent over the entire reunion episode.

Avoidance through neutral ignoring (A2). Subtle signs of feeling. The child may greet the parent, orient to the parent, and at times respond or reply to the parent. The child may even initiate a greeting, though careful study of the greeting will indicate that it may actually be an effort to get past the necessary niceties (e.g., a dismissing, sing-song, "HEL-lo"). The child may briefly query the parent but remains busy with other activities, which remain foremost. Neutral ignoring of the parent is the most striking characteristic of the episode, but subtle and non-confrontational signs of anger and annoyance may be present. Sometimes the child may "warm" to the parent slightly by the very end of the reunion episode, as do infants placed in Ainsworth's more moderately avoidant (A2) infancy sub-classification.

Insecure-Ambivalent (Group C)

As in infancy, this is the most heterogeneous group of children. Initially, our judges worked only with the three major classifications identified above, but three of four children who had been ambivalent were identified through failure to fit to the secure, insecure-avoidant, or insecure-directing criteria. Two of these children (classified C2, or ambivalent-passive in infancy) were identified by the judge as resembling one another, while not resembling the other children in the sample. A third (classified as C1, or ambivalent-actively resistant in infancy) was judged to resemble one of the C2 children, but on the whole to be unlike any other child in the sample. The behavior of all four children was considered incoherent.

In infancy, insecure-ambivalent children are identified by their distress, by fearfulness regarding the unfamiliar environment or the stranger, and through their weak to strong proximity-seeking toward the parent combined with weak to strong resistance and anger. In addition, the insecure-ambivalent infant is marked by an inability to be "settled" by the parent.

Insecure-ambivalent children at 6 years of age show moderate avoidance, mixed with or eventually supplanted by direct looks and direct responses to the parent. Because the child may talk to the parent with the back turned to the parent; move away from the parent, then smile and interact in a manner which is simultaneously pleasant and avoidant; or exhibit smooth, neutral avoidance suddenly interrupted by initiating clearly ambivalent physical contact, the avoidance is not usual in its form nor (when it ends) in its sequelae.

The behavior of the insecure-ambivalent 6-year-old is distinctly confusing, since there are likely to be elements of avoidance, sadness, subtle fear, and subtle to open hostility. These mixed indices of insecurity are likely to be combined with immature behavior, such as "cute" whininess, "cute" affectionateness, "cute" proximity-seeking or contact-seeking in which physical ambivalence about proximity to the parent is striking.

These children cannot be classified as insecure-avoidant because their avoidance is not strong enough, or, if strong, is not well organized. They cannot be classified as insecure-directing because their hostile behavior is either simple and direct without being directing, or is indirect and bizarre. They cannot be classified as secure (e.g., secure-reserved, for moderate avoidance) because of subtle indices of fear, ambivalent movements when near the parent, looks of sadness, or indices of disorganization. In addition, the child's "cute" behavior, and the form taken by its occasional immature whininess is incompatible with a sense of security with the parent.

There are two sub-classifications:

Ambivalent-hostile (C1). The child shows moderate avoidance of the parent, combined with some hostility. The hostility may be expressed immediately but does not seem part of an effort to control the parent or the situation or to humiliate or embarrass the parent. One boy in our sample said immediately upon father's entrance, suddenly and loudly, "AND . . . the little boy is dead! . . . AND, the little girl is dead!" He then threw himself upon the stuffed lion, kicking his legs, and then added, "AND . . . the little baby is dead, too." He then responded normally, although in a whiny voice, whenever addressed by the parent. At one moment, he showed a definite fear-face. In addition, there were several moments of genuine mutual smiling and warmth between the child and his father.

Ambivalent-passive (C2). There are indices of sadness and disorganization in this child, and perhaps looks of surprise and confusion at the parent's entrance. There is some avoidance (neutral avoidance, or even moving immediately away), but also definite efforts to fit into what is perhaps expected by the parent – pseudo-bright smiles, wriggling or gingerly approaches, contact and or proximity-seeking. The child seems to be attempting to appear at ease, but there is an underlying sense that the child is "acting." Faintly lost, angry, or apprehensive looks appear upon slow-motion study of the tape.

One child in our sample initially moved away from the mother, then lay on her stomach beside her, wriggling uncomfortably and talking in a breathy "baby" voice. When she sat up to speak with her mother, she cocked her head to the side, as though attempting to be engaging. Finally, she put her arm around her mother's shoulders, although in a gingerly manner. While simultaneously pulling away from mother, she kept her arm around her shoulder and attempted to point out various objects in the room (as though 'teaching' the mother).

Another child looked distressed and dropped down behind a piece of furniture immediately upon mother's entrance, then straightened up with a look of surprise, as though he had just realized mother was within the room. This child seemed to be *acting* whenever he looked at the mother, looking directly several times into mother's face with a tight, bright, "toothy" smile. When mother was not looking at him, however, he sometimes looked at her apprehensively, or with subtle resentment. His behavior throughout the episode was smooth.

Caveats

With so few "C" infants available for the first Berkeley sample, we risk making universal rules out of incidental correlates. There may be some children who should be classified insecure-ambivalent at six who are not substantially avoidant.

There is no question that some of the behaviors mentioned are seen in children whose correct classification is, for example, secure or insecure-avoidant. Head-cocking, use of a childish voice, and some cute behavior occurred in several non-C children in the Berkeley sample. None of these are signs of "C" in itself. These correlated behaviors are important chiefly in terms of the evidence they provide for a fairly consistent effort on the child's part to act some kind of a role.

While the avoidant child seems to pretend to independence and occasionally maturity, the ambivalent child seems to pretend to relatedness and/or the state of dependence upon the parent.

Insecure-Controlling/Directing (Group D)

These children have openly or subtly taken control of the child–parent relationship. In the Berkeley laboratory, children judged insecure-directing at six had been judged insecure-disorganized (see Main & Solomon, 1986) in infancy. As noted earlier, this initial disorganization may be the result of disorganization of the parental caregiving system, itself a result of attachment-related trauma occurring before the parent had reached adulthood.

Our studies indicate, however, that an infant does not remain simply disorganized: Rather, it comes to assume some control within the relationship. At six, there is role-reversal, taking one of two forms. The child (1) may take confrontational control of the parent, treating her punitively, acting to embarrass her, or openly rejecting her and ordering her to leave or move away. Or, the child may seem to subtly attempt to (2) take care of the parent, either through overly bright greetings and attempts to cheer the parent or through more directly guiding and orienting caregiving behavior and helpfully orienting and directing her. In addition, there may still be some direct though subtle signs of behavioral disorganization.

Directing-Punitive (D1)

The child acts to humiliate, embarrass, or reject the parent. This may occur at the moment of the parent's entrance into the room, when the parent is openly, confrontationally ignored or rejected. The child may indicate a wish for the parent not to return to the room (e.g., "Don't bother me!"), or a wish for the parent to leave the room (e.g., "I am NOT going – why don't you leave!"). The child may make humiliating, embarrassing, or belittling remarks to the parent (e.g., "You're really clumsy, ha-ha!"; "Sit down and keep your eyes closed."; "I told you, keep quiet!"). The child may refuse to leave the room with the parent.

The punitive-directing child may also reject the parent through "punitive silence," a silence that is so timed as to leave the parent humiliated and embarrassed. This can be done by simply waiting a few seconds too long to respond to direct parental queries, e.g., "What are you doing, honey?", ". . . playing"; or by failing to respond at all.

Punitive silence can be distinguished from ignoring, in that it is humiliating or embarrassing to the parent, and hence directly rejecting and confrontational. The child does not "cover" for its silence, hence saving face for the parent, but fails to respond in a manner that embarrasses the parent. (Avoidant ignoring may also involve silences, but these are so placed that they can be ignored in turn by the parent without humiliation or embarrassment).

Directing-Caregiving (D2)

The child may show an overly bright greeting and may attempt to cheer the parent. Or, the child may help the parent or helpfully direct the parent's attention during the reunion episode. This behavior is subtle, and may be difficult to distinguish initially from security. Here, we offer examples of both the initial, over-bright greeting (seen in some, but not all of these children) and helpful, cheering, and directing behavior. Note that a child may be classified as "caregiving" if she shows *either* of these patterns.

Overly Bright Behavior (D2a)

The child's greeting is extremely positive, and indeed brighter than that of children judged "very secure" with the parent. Study of behavior just prior to the greeting, and/or just following it, however, indicates its insecure quality. One child in the Berkeley sample had been in the playroom with the mother (with whom she was secure), when she heard the father returning. She said to the mother, in an unmistakably depressed and resigned tone, "He's coming," but then immediately upon reunion gave an exceptionally bright greeting and smile, ("DAD!"), and began immediately to attempt to direct and guide her father's attention ("See, this is a . . .").

Another child in the Berkeley sample showed a sudden, startling change in behavior and movement on the appearance of the mother, as though the appearance of the mother had a disorganizing or disrupting effect upon behavior. Initially, we attributed this change entirely to the child's delight in seeing the parent, since he smiled extremely broadly, his upper torso almost "jerking" forward toward the parent. This child said, "MOM!–chee!–wow!", as though exclaiming upon the reappearance of the parent. Immediately following this extreme greeting, the child's face became affectless, and he turned to play with the castle. The remainder of the episode had a quality of subtle avoidance. We see this behavior as caregiving because the child seems to be assuming responsibility for uplifting, elevating, or maintaining the parent's mood.

Finally, two children ran to the door upon reunion as though delighted and seeking contact, and then immediately turned away from the door with a confused expression. One of the children put hand to mouth as though in apprehension as she turned away. These particular behavior patterns – termed *disordering of expected temporal sequences,* and *direct indices of confusion or apprehension* – are also seen in infancy in children judged insecure-disorganized.

Insecure-Directing: Caregiving (D2b)

Like overly bright behavior, this has a positive quality, which also may initially be taken for security. The child is unusually helpful and solicitous toward the parent, demonstrating concern or care in a manner suggesting the parent is dependent upon the child for guidance.

One child moved directly to the parent, hugging her (while holding her body slightly away from her): "*Mommy* . . . I *love* you." At other times, indices of role-reversing efforts to cheer or direct the parent are shown in speech alone. "Want to play with me, mommy, in the sandbox? . . . It's fun, isn't it, mommy?". "Daddy, you're making such a wonderful castle – isn't he, mommy?". The child may also attempt helpfully to direct the attention of a flustered, disorganized parent: "Look at this, now, daddy. This one here. That's right, this one." The tone of the child's voice is likely to be solicitous and protective.

Caveats

We see children who are placed in the over-bright and in the controlling-caregiving categories as attempting to alter the parent's mood or state, or else to help the parent maintain positive aspects of his or her state of the moment. These children can be exquisitely sensitive to the parent's mood, and their behaviors can be solely positive. Nonetheless, this can be seen as inappropriate. Behavior of this kind is observed in abused children and in children of depressed mothers.

Since the behavior of consistently over-bright and/or caregiving children can be wholly bright, sensitive, and positive, it can be difficult to distinguish (a) from the behavior of children who are genuinely this way and (b) from the behavior of children who simply sense that, at this particular moment, the parent is down or distressed – and who attempt, correspondingly and only temporarily, to cheer. In attempting to distinguish, it may be helpful to look especially carefully at the child's pre-entrance behavior. What we are looking for is over-bright or caregiving behavior which appears *immediately* at the "thought" of the parent – that is, which is built into the relationship – rather than any which might appear in response to a later perception that the parent is somewhat down today. Brightness and caregiving of this kind do not merely alleviate the parent's present but temporary depression or anxiety, but ultimately are used to relieve or to forestall the experience of anxiety by the child.

Insecure-Unclassified

We suggest that the sixth-year classification system be left open for further description and development. We have found several children for whom none of the A, B, C, or D categories seemed to fit. These have necessarily to be termed "insecure-unclassified." In addition, some coherent new categories may be emerging. One of the latter can best be described as *sexualized.* Another possible candidate is a child who appeared so depressed as to be unable to participate in social interactions with the parent.

As an example of insecure-unclassified, one child seemed nervous and shy at the return of the mother, stammering and twisting his arms together. His behavior from the beginning of the episode seemed that of a child who feels inadequate and shy, in the presence of a teacher who is the object of a "crush". Later, this child made mildly sexually suggestive remarks and movements, while still appearing nervous. This behavior pattern did not fit any of the developed categories.

At present, we are distinguishing between children who seem *sexualized* in relationship to the parent and children who simply seem insecure in ways not yet systematically specified. A child who simply seemed nervous or depressed, without being avoidant, ambivalent, or directing would be placed in the category.

References

Ainsworth, M.D.S. (1984). Personal communication, May.

Ainsworth, M.D.S. (1985). Personal communication, January.

Ainsworth, M.D.S., Bell, S.M., & Stayton, D.J. (1971). Individual differences in strange-situation behaviour of one-year-olds. In H.R. Schaffer (Eds.), *The Origins of Human Social Relations* (pp. 17–58). London and New York: Academic Press.

Ainsworth, M.D.S., Blehar, M.C., Waters, E., & Wall, S. (1978). *Patterns of Attachment: A Psychological Study of the Strange Situation*. Hillsdale, NJ: Erlbaum.

Ainsworth, M.D.S., & Eichberg, C.G. (1991). Effects of infant mother attachment of mothers' unresolved loss of an attachment figure or other traumatic experiences. In C. Parkes, J. Stevenson-Hinde, & P. Marris (Eds.), *Attachment Across the Life Cycle* (pp. 160–183). New York: Routledge.

Ainsworth, M.D.S., & Wittig, B.A. (1969). Attachment and exploratory behavior of one-year-olds in a strange situation. In B.M. Foss (Ed.), *Determinants of Infant Behavior* (Vol. 4, pp. 113–136). London: Methuen.

Arend, R., Gove, F.L., & Sroufe, L.A. (1979). Continuity of individual adaptation from infancy to kindergarten: A predictive study of ego-resiliency and curiosity in preschoolers. *Child Development, 50*, 950–959.

Bowlby, J. (1969). *Attachment and Loss. Vol. 1. Attachment*. New York: Basic Books.

Bowlby, J. (1973). *Attachment and Loss. Vol. 2. Separation: Anxiety and Anger*. New York: Basic Books.

Bowlby, J. (1980). *Attachment and Loss. Vol. 3. Loss: Sadness & Depression*. London: Hogarth Press.

Bowlby, J. (1990). *Letter to Sonia Monteiro de Barros*. London: Wellcome Archive.

Bretherton, I. (1985). Attachment theory: Retrospect and prospect. *Monographs of the Society for Research in Child Development, 50*, 3.

Bretherton, I., & Ainsworth, M.D.S. (1974). Responses of one-year-olds to a stranger in a strange situation. In M. Lewis & L.A. Rosenblum (Eds.), *The Origin of Fear* (pp. 134–164). New York: Wiley.

Crittenden, P.M. (1985). Maltreated infants: Vulnerability and resilience. *Journal of Child Psychology and Psychiatry, 26*, 85–96.

Crittenden, P.M., & DiLalla, D.L. (1988). Compulsive compliance: The development of an inhibitory coping strategy in infancy. *Journal of Abnormal Child Psychology, 16*(5), 585–599.

Crowell, J.A, & Feldman, S.S. (1988). Mothers' internal models of relationships and children's behavioral and developmental status: A study of mother-child interaction. *Child Development, 59*, 1273–1285.

Egeland, B., & Sroufe, L.A. (1981a). Attachment and early maltreatment. *Child Development, 52*, 44–52.

Egeland, B., & Sroufe, L.A. (1981b). Developmental sequelae of maltreatment in infancy. In D. Cicchetti & R. Rizley (Eds.), *Developmental Perspectives in Child Maltreatment* (pp. 77–92). San Francisco: Jossey Bass.

Eichberg, C.G. (1987). *Quality of infant-parent attachment: Related to mother's representation of her own relationship history and child care attitudes*. Unpublished doctoral dissertation, University of Virginia. [See Ainsworth & Eichberg, (1991)].

Fremmer-Bombik, E. (1986). Unpublished doctoral thesis, Regensburg University, Germany. See Grossman, K. et al. (1988).

Friedman, C.T. (1986). *Interaction and attachment: Determinants of individual differences in a sample of visually impaired one and two-year-olds and their mothers*. Unpublished doctoral dissertation, University of California, Berkeley.

Gaensbauer, T.J., & Harmon, R.J. (1982). Attachment behaviour in abused/neglected and premature infants: Implications for the concept of attachment. In R.N. Emde & R.J. Harmon (Eds.), *The Attachment and Affiliative Systems* (pp. 263–280). New York: Plenum Press.

George, C. (1984). *Individual differences in affective sensitivity: A study of five-year olds and their parents*. Unpublished doctoral dissertation, University of California, Berkeley.

George, C., Kaplan, N., & Main, M. (1985). *An adult attachment interview: Interview protocol*. Unpublished manuscript, University of California, Berkeley.

George, C., & Main, M. (1979). Social interactions of young abused children: Approach, avoidance and aggression. *Child Development, 58*, 306–318.

Goodnow, J.J. (1977). *Children's Drawings*. London: Fontana.

Greenberg, M., Cichetti, D., & Cummings, M. (1990). *Attachment in the Preschool Years: Theory, Research, and Intervention*. Chicago: University of Chicago Press.

Grossmann, K., Fremmer-Bombik, E., Rudolph, J., & Grossmann, K.E. (1988). Maternal attachment representations as related to patterns of infant–mother attachment and maternal care during the first year. In R.A. Hinde & J. Stevenson-Hinde (Eds.), *Relationships within Families* (pp. 241–260). Oxford: Oxford Science Publications.

Hinde, R. (1982). Attachment: Some conceptual and biological issues. In C. Parkes & J. Stevenson-Hinde (Eds.), *The Place of Attachment in Human Behaviour* (pp. 60–76). New York: Basic Books.

Kaplan, N. (1987). *Individual differences in six-year-olds' thoughts about separation: Predicted to actual experiences of separation*. Unpublished doctoral dissertation, University of California, Berkeley.

Kaplan, N., & Main, M. (1986). *Assessment of attachment organisation through children's family drawings*. Unpublished manuscript Department of Psychology, University of California, Berkeley.

Kobak, R., & Sceery, A. (1988). Attachment in late adolescence: Working models, affect regulation, and representations of self and others. *Child Development, 59*, 135–146.

Krentz, M.S. (1982). *Qualitative differences between mother-child and caregiver-child attachments of infants in family daycare*. Unpublished doctoral dissertation, the California School of Professional Psychology, Berkeley.

Main, M. (1981). Avoidance in the service of attachment: A working paper. In K. Immelman, G.W. Barlow, L. Petrinovich, & M. Main (Eds.), *Behavioural Development: The Bielefeld Interdisciplinary Project*. New York: Cambridge University Press.

Main, M. (1983). Exploration, play, and cognitive functioning related to infant-mother attachment. *Infant Behavior and Development, 6*, 167–174.

Main, M., & Cassidy, J. (1988). Categories of response to reunion with the parent at age 6: Predictable from infant attachment classifications and stable over a 1-month period. *Developmental Psychology, 24*, 415–426.

Main, M., & Hesse, E. (1990). Parents' unresolved traumatic experiences are related to infant disorganized attachment status: Is Frightened and/or frightening parental behavior the linking mechanism? In M. Greenberg, D. Cicchetti, & M. Cummings (Eds.), *Attachment in the Preschool Years* (pp. 161–182). Chicago: University of Chicago Press.

Main, M., Kaplan, N., & Cassidy, J. (1985). Security in infancy, childhood and adulthood: A move to the level of representation. In I. Bretherton & E. Waters (Eds.), *Growing Points in Attachment Theory*. Research Monographs of the Society for Research in Child Development 50 (1–2, Serial No. 209) (pp. 66–104). Chicago: University of Chicago Press.

Main, M., & Solomon, J. (1986). Discovery of an insecure-disorganized/disoriented attachment pattern. In T.B. Brazelton & M.W. Yogman (Eds.), *Affective Development in Infancy* (pp. 95–124). Norwood, NJ: Ablex Publishing.

Main, M., & Solomon, J. (1990). Procedures for identifying infants as disorganized/disoriented during the Ainsworth Strange Situation. In M. Greenberg, D. Cicchetti, & M. Cummings (Eds.), *Attachment in the Preschool Years: Theory, Research, and Intervention* (pp. 121–160). Chicago: University of Chicago Press.

Main, M., & Stadtman, J. (1981). Infant response to rejection of physical contact by the mother: Aggression avoidance and conflict. *Journal of American Academy of Child Psychiatry, 20*, 292–307.

Main, M., & Weston, D. (1981). The quality of the toddler's relationship to mother and father judged to differ in security. *Child Development, 52*, 932–940.

Main, M., & Weston, D. (1982). Avoidance of the attachment figure in infancy: Descriptions and interpretations. In C.M. Parkes & J. Stevenson-Hinde (Eds.), *The Place of Attachment in Human Behaviour*. London: Tavistock Publications.

Matas, L., Arend, R.A., & Sroufe, L.A. (1978). Continuity of adaptation in the second year: The relationship between quality of attachment and later competence. *Child Development, 49*, 547–556.

Mayr, E. (1976). *Evolution and the Diversity of Life: Selected Essays*. Cambridge, MA: Belknap Press.

Solomon, J., George, C., & Ivins, B. (1987, April). *Mother-child interaction in the home and security of attachment at age six*. Paper presented at the biennial meeting of the Society for Research in Child Development, Baltimore, MD.

Spieker, S.J., & Booth, C. (1985). Family risk typologies and patterns of insecure attachment. In J.O. Osofsky (Chair), *Intervention with infants at risk: Patterns of attachment*. Symposium conducted at the Biennial Meeting of the Society for Research in Child Development, Toronto, April 27.

Sroufe, L.A. (1983). Infant-caregiver attachment and patterns of adaptation in preschool: The roots of maladaptation and competence. In M. Perlmutter (Ed.), *Minnesota Symposium in Child Psychology* (Vol. 16, pp. 41–81). Hillsdale, NJ: Erlbaum.

Sroufe, L.A., & Waters, E. (1977). Attachment as an organisational construct. *Child Development, 48*, 1184–1199.

Strage, A., & Main, M. (1985). Parent child discourse patterns at six years predicted from the organisation of infant attachment relationships. In M. Main (Chair), *Attachment: A move to the level of representation*. Biannual meeting of the Society for Research in Child Development, Toronto, Canada, April.

Trivers, R.L. (1974). Parent-offspring conflict. *American Zoologist, 14*, 249–264.

Vaughn, B., Egeland, B., Sroufe, L.A., & Waters E. (1979). Individual differences in infant-mother attachment at twelve and eighteen months: Stability and change in families under stress. *Child Development, 50*, 971–975.

Wartner, U.G. (1987). *Attachment in infancy and at age six and children's self-concepts: A follow-up of a German longitudinal study*. Unpublished doctoral dissertation, University of Virginia.

Wartner, U.G., Grossmann, K., Fremmer-Bombik, E., & Suess, G. (1994). Attachment patterns at age six in South Germany: Predictability from infancy and implications for preschool behavior. *Child Development, 65*, 1014–1027.

Waters, E. (1978). The reliability and stability of individual differences in infant-mother attachment. *Child Development, 49*(2), 483–494.

Waters, E., Wippmann, J., & Sroufe, L.A. (1979). Attachment, positive affect, and competence in the peer group: Two studies in construct validation. *Child Development, 50*(3), 821–829.

Index

Note: page numbers in *italics* indicate a figure, page numbers in **bold** indicate a table, and page numbers followed by an 'n' indicate a note on the corresponding page.

For Product Safety Concerns and Information please contact our EU
representative GPSR@taylorandfrancis.com
Taylor & Francis Verlag GmbH, Kaufingerstraße 24, 80331 München, Germany

www.ingramcontent.com/pod-product-compliance
Lightning Source LLC
LaVergne TN
LVHW020343240926
848761LV00033B/291

* 9 7 8 1 0 3 2 9 3 7 2 4 3 *